# Troubled Voices

# Troubled Voices

Stories of Ethics and Illness

*Richard M. Zaner*

The Pilgrim Press

Cleveland, Ohio

The Pilgrim Press, Cleveland, Ohio 44115
© 1993 by Richard M. Zaner

These characters are based on composite cases and names have been
changed to protect privacy

98   97   96   95   94          5   4   3   2

Library of Congress Cataloging-in-Publication Data
Zaner, Richard M.
Troubled voices : stories of ethics and illness / Richard M. Zaner.
p.   cm.
Includes bibliographical references and index.
ISBN 0-8298-0964-3 (acid-free paper)
1. Medical ethics—Case studies.
2. Hospitals—Moral and ethical aspects.   I. Title.
R724.Z36   1993
174′ .2—dc20
93-3823
CIP

*For June,*
*my love, for knowing that*
*what I thought impossible,*
*then improbable, could be done*
*and was worth it*
*after all.*

# Contents

❖

# Foreword

A quarter of a century ago medical ethics was *terra incognita* for most philosophers. They saw it as a minor branch of ethics, essentially a set of moral assertions without a formal conceptual framework. Moreover, medical ethics was an "applied" field and *ipso facto* low on the pecking order of academic respectability. Physicians for their part felt no need for philosophical assistance. Armed with the Hippocratic oath and a long tradition of ethical commitment, they could not envision how any resident of the "ivory tower," much less a philosopher, could possibly help them in the urgent and complex dilemmas they had to face daily.

Despite these negative signals from both relevant disciplines, a few philosophers became intrigued by the ethical and philosophical dilemmas that medicine had begun to encounter in the middle sixties of this century. They sensed that the unprecedented expansion of medical technology, the improvement of public education, and the growth of participatory democracy with the civil rights and consumer movements were creating ethical problems that would challenge the structures of traditional medical ethics. They perceived too that the newer and more complex ethical problems would have to be resolved in a morally pluralistic society whose moral moorings in the Jewish and Christian faiths had been seriously weakened.

For these few prescient philosophers the need for a formal and systematic inquiry into the conceptual framework of medical ethics was obvious. Their foresight has since been amply confirmed. Today philosophers are everywhere immersed in every aspect of the theoretical and practical problems of medical ethics. Their influence has transformed it from the private preserve of the medical profession into the most intensely and widely debated branch of moral philosophy.

Richard Zaner, whose reflections we are privileged to read in this book, was one of the more intrepid of those few philosophers bold enough to become involved with medicine in the sixties. He was, and remains, a thoroughly qualified phenomenologist who has brought his philosophical insight to bear fruitfully on the philosophy of medicine as well as its ethics. Zaner first became intrigued with medicine when he accepted an appointment to teach philosophy and ethics to medical students at the new Health Sciences Center I was establishing at the State University of New York at Stony Brook. He moved directly from academic philosophy to teaching students in the health professions and interacting with their clinical and basic science instruction. In recent years, in the Department of Medicine at Vanderbilt where he now holds a chair in medical ethics, he has expanded these interests into the hospital and clinical arena.

In the hospital, Zaner has acted as consultant, counselor, and friend to patients, families, physicians, and nurses. Through a series of clinical cases in which he participated, he narrates his experiences in rich detail in this book. The reader of what Zaner calls his clinical "stories" is afforded a privileged insight into the singular personal odyssey of a philosopher who remains a philosopher, but who has now become a genuine clinician as well.

Zaner's reflections reveal the intellectual and psychological transformation he experienced as he confronted the world of the hospital. Repeatedly, with genuine humility and probing introspection, Zaner asked himself: What am I doing here? How can a philosopher possibly help? How can *I* help? There were no precedents to guide him. He encountered puzzlement and skepticism among the clinicians who asked him for help. These clinicians were not sure how a "phenomenologist" could be useful at the bedside of all places. Nonetheless, they sensed their need for assistance and consulted him. In these narratives, Zaner explores the answers to his own and his colleagues' questions.

With each tale, Zaner reveals how he could, indeed, be helpful to his clinical colleagues. The wide range of cases in which clinicians sought his assistance speaks eloquently to his capacity to help—from the neonatal and obstetrical service through the dialysis unit to genetic counseling, HIV infection, and transplantation surgery. Zaner's success in gaining the respect and confidence of such a wide range of clinicians is most impressive. It is certainly not the universal experience of all ethicists who venture on hospital floors.

These stories have intrinsic human interest on their own. But they also have much to teach clinicians and ethicists about how best to bridge the gap between philosophical speculation and clinical decision making. What comes through in every case is Zaner's felicitous combination of personal qualities and his special style of philosophizing. This combination is central to his success in communicating with the clinicians, their patients, and the patients' families in a nonthreatening, open, and helpful way.

Zaner clearly is no reformer intent on rescuing medicine and its practitioners from their moral failings. Nor is he content to be the rational analyst of ethical principles and conflicts from the outside. Too often ethicists who have attempted to play such roles have generated a serious backlash that defeated any help they might have been able to provide. Instead, Zaner approached his new challenges with genuine humility and honest skepticism about what he might contribute. Although he was intellectually intrigued by the clinical dilemmas he encountered, he had respect for their urgency and complexity. He did not fancy himself the delegated intellect whose role it was to enlighten clinicians, to bring order into their thinking, or to safeguard patients from clinical paternalism. But when needed,

Zaner provided these—but always by gentle, respectful indirection and with the conviction that he was learning along with those he counseled.

Married to Zaner's personal qualities and, indeed, intrinsic to them is his personal view of philosophy and philosophizing. This he delineated in *The Way of Phenomenology,* [1] published in 1970 just as he undertook his engagement with medicine for the first time at Stony Brook.

In the prologue to that book, Zaner says that "philosophy is essentially this activity of questioning and pondering that is dialogue." [2] But the aim of the dialogue is not to give opinion, as so many ethicists and those who consult them believe. Rather, for Zaner, dialogue is a form of communication that imposes certain duties upon the questioner

> to listen to all responses, to be responsive to would-be answers,
> and to make sure, through further critical questions, that I
> fully understand and assess the responses. As a responder, I bear
> a coordinate responsibility to respond responsibly and to
> recognize and accept responsively the responsibility of answer-
> ing and of being open, to explain, clarify, and, if need be, to
> defend my responses before the one who questions. [3]

Zaner consistently puts this idea of philosophizing to work in his communication with patients, families, and those who attend them medically. In his narration of each case, he makes it clear that he is immersed in a common quest with those who seek his help. His aim is not to display his technical proficiency as an ethicist, but through questions and responses to enable others to see what course of action is best for them. Zaner strives to put himself in the other person's shoes—a simple way to express the aim of his finely honed and sophisticated use of dialogue.

It is a pleasure, and genuinely instructive, to see how Zaner's innate compassion and empathy, his gentle skepticism about his own capabilities, his humility, and his special view of the philosopher's task interact with each other. Other ethicists have been successful at the bedside using other methods, but none more successful than Zaner.

It is a privilege to be privy to this internal reflection of a true philosopher who maintains his identity as a philosopher even in the clinical setting and through that identity helps others in the midst of the anxiety, suffering, and urgency of making moral choices. Zaner's odyssey has much to teach philosophers, health professionals, and families about the humanization of the predicaments of illness and healing.

Edmund D. Pellegrino, M.D.
Director, Center for the Advanced Study of Ethics
Georgetown University

# Acknowledgments

❖

Writing this book has been a continuous learning experience. I have been a university professor for the past thirty-three years and have been involved as an ethicist and philosopher in the world of medicine and health care for the past twenty-two. In many ways, I have learned much about philosophy and ethics from my students in philosophy, medicine, religious studies, and other fields, as I have from my many clinical encounters with health professionals, patients, families, and others. Their kindness is gratefully acknowledged.

Out of respect for the people whose lives and challenges inspired this book, I decided to make these narratives my own inventions; their lives, voices, and troubles, along with countless others in the over twenty years of my involvement in this field, formed only the basis for these stories. I must nevertheless acknowledge my profound gratitude to the many people—patients and their families and friends, physicians, nurses, and other providers—who have been so generous, perhaps unwittingly, in helping me understand what they were going through during moments of illness and crisis. The courage, honesty, and wisdom these people showed as they struggled with difficult medical and moral issues are a constant source of wonder and hope. Despite so much said nowadays about the "decay" of moral life in our society, my encounters with these people persuade me that things are not as awful as we oftentimes hear.

Several people have gladly given their time, insight, and enthusiasm as this project began to take shape from its very tentative beginnings over ten years ago. A dear friend for many years and a wonderfully caring physician, Eric Cassell read several early versions of the manuscript, offering numerous important suggestions. Edmund D. Pellegrino—whose vision, learning, and incredible energy almost singled-handedly brought about the fields of medical humanities and clinical ethics—first got me involved in these issues and has been a close friend ever since. Ed not only read an earlier version of the manuscript, but to my utter delight agreed to write a prefatory word for it.

Finally, I am deeply indebted to the sound editorial sense and sheer labor devoted to this project by Marian ("Shug") McBay, a senior fellow in Clinical and Research Ethics at The Center for Clinical and Research Ethics at Vanderbilt University Medical Center. She brought intelligence and imagination to the project and was a constant, strong voice encouraging me to commit to the doing of the thing. Her ability to get inside these stories, to appreciate their rhythm and direction, is simply remarkable—working with her has been an altogether delightful and rewarding experience for me.

None of these fine people should be held responsible for the book, of course, although, truth be told, their help and encouragement has surely made it far finer than it would otherwise have been.

# Prologue

This book is somewhat unusual; and because it is, some comment is in order. In what follows, I relate some of the experiences I've had since becoming rather deeply involved in trying to help people—patients and families and friends, physicians, nurses, and others working in hospitals—deal with the problems they face during times of illness, injury, or the consequences of handicap, whether from genetic, congenital, or social circumstances. What I do has come to be termed "clinical ethics," and I am often referred to as an "ethicist." I didn't invent these terms; in fact, early on in my involvement I actively resisted both. The first, because I wasn't at all convinced that there was a place for a philosopher in clinical settings; the second, because it smacks of a sort of "expert," a label that few, if any, of us in this field want to claim. But the terms are already in wide currency in the health professions, like it or not, and, I suppose, I've had to learn to make my peace with that fact.

So, over the past decade or so I've come to be known as an "ethicist." It is certainly okay to wonder what in the world that means, to expect some sort of answer from me. In what follows, I try to give some response to that question, for, in a way, I decided to share these stories in an effort to get clear on that for myself. What better way to say what an ethicist is than to tell the story of how I happened to become one? I say "become," for that is just about what occurred: I surely did not set out years ago with that as my aim. When I first became involved in the realm of the health professions in 1971, it didn't occur to me then, or to anyone else I knew, that any of us would be doing the sort of thing I've wound up doing for the past ten years.

It didn't even occur to me, with much clarity anyway, that I would become more than just an interested observer when a decade ago I asked physicians whether I could trail along with them on many of their daily clinical rounds. They were not only gracious enough to allow me to do that, but gradually I found myself being asked to *help*, though it was hardly clear to anyone, me least of all, just how or whether I could actually help. It was only through the course of being involved, being asked to help and trying to be responsive to these requests, that this peculiar form of work began to get clearer. Slowly, I began to discover something like the idea, even a definition, of what I was engaged in.

While it is not unreasonable to ask, here, about that idea, I'd like to hold off on that. I recall what one of my philosophy professors said in a class years ago: "definitions should come only *after* the work of discovery; if you start out with them, you'll most likely end up more obscuring important things than elucidating them." Or something like that. His point, I think, was that the experience of discovery is a vital part of "getting the idea." In any event, it has seemed to me that the voyage—from shaky, tentative beginnings to something firmer—is both more interesting and, hopefully, more inviting than a polemical exposition. So, while I do not want to leave that matter entirely up in the air, my aim is to take you through some part of my own recent history, these stories, where I came to understand more about clinical ethics and being an ethicist. Realizing this carries with it a certain burden, I have to ask your forbearance and patience while I make my way through some key experiences that I hope will sharpen—both make clearer, and give a keen edge to—our appreciation of the crucial place of ethical considerations in clinical encounters.

Ethics has become something of a buzzword these days and for that very reason is in danger of becoming confused and obscure. Its very frequency of use threatens to erode its solid sense, rather like hard rock worn by rushing water. You hear someone complain that an athlete "took unfair advantage" of competitors by using steroids; but aside from the damage done to the athlete's own body and soul, most of us may be hard pressed to say just what we mean by "unfair." Our electoral system is often said to favor the rich, and we hear that it is just not "right"; but what we mean, or are supposed to mean, by this may not in turn be at all obvious. And we are fairly deluged with arguments about the "welfare system"; yet, if we wonder about the meaning of that, of the "good" of the common weal, many of us feel little short of stumped.

When it comes to the field of health care, our daily media are crammed with item after item that even slight notice suggests is somehow "ethical" (or "unethical," since that's the way the word is so often used nowadays). From abortion to "pulling the plug," from "test-tube babies" to "playing God," from "inventing new life forms" to "exorbitant costs"—our ethics menu is jam-packed, so full that few of us can comprehend the scope and reach of what medicine and biomedical science have increasingly made available in our society. For all the apparent benefits we reap with burgeoning new technologies, however, our infant mortality rate remains dismal (an infant born in Harlem has less chance to survive to her teens than one born in many so-called third-world nations). Although we currently spend more than 13 percent of our GNP on health care, a large amount goes to keeping people merely alive, to merely prolonging dying (currently, about one billion dollars is spent on the last six months of life), which seems at best unwise and at worst inhumane, as any of us knows full well when we ourselves have to suffer through the protracted and painful dying of a hopelessly ill loved one.

But what is it like to *be* in situations like these? What are things like from the point of view of the people who face giving birth to a severely ill and damaged baby? What is it like for a person who is terminally ill and only a single-lung or heart transplant can stay that grisly prospect? What is it really like to be an old person whose heart, lungs, and kidneys are failing but who desperately wants to stay alive if only for a time to see grandchildren or a dear old friend once again? And what is it like to be gravely ill but uninsured and with no hope for help?

To be involved in clinical ethics is to meet people like this, people who for whatever reason find themselves on the edge, at the bottom, utterly focused and trapped by their sick bodies or minds. It is also to meet their families and friends, each of whom has, or would like to have, some voice in decisions that have to be made. And, it is to meet still other people who profess the ability to help the sick and maimed get better: doctors, nurses, social workers, chaplains, therapists, dietitians, technicians—the host of people in the halls and wards and rooms of hospitals, nursing homes, hospices, rehab facilities, even home health-care settings. All these meetings, we are quickly forced to realize, go on within a penumbra of written and unwritten rules, regulations, policies, statutes, federal and state procedures, and innumerable legal decisions. They go on within our particular society with its history, traditions, norms, social values, mores, and folkways. Meeting sick people, families, and providers turns out to be terrifically complicated. Add to that the fact that for the most part all these different people are *strangers* to each other; and when trust is most problematic yet most needed, we are forced to realize just how ripe clinical situations are for conflicts, dilemmas, problems, even downright enigmas when it comes, as it ineluctably always does, to the business of making decisions everyone hopes are right, good, and fair.

Clinical ethics concerns that complex of relationships: doctor/patient, nurse/patient, doctor/nurse, patient/hospital, doctor/hospital, patient/family, state law/patient condition, and on and on. Just what, where, how, and why always depend on the specific circumstances of the patient and diagnosis, but also on matters we often don't like to think about, such as how much and what type of insurance, what sort of hospital we may be taken to after an accident, and what policies it has and which values it embodies. Finding out what we have to pay attention to is a matter, most often, of plain talk. As one of my favorite physicians, and a good friend, likes to say, "language is the most important tool the physician has." However this works out in clinical medicine, it is surely true of clinical ethics, for, ultimately, making decisions is a matter of helping the people who must make the decisions to figure out, in any specific set of circumstances, what is most deeply cherished by and worthwhile for *them,* the people who are ill, those who care for them, and those who take care of them. To do this, people have to talk, discuss, converse, which is not easy for them to do with the difficulties they face.

Clinical ethics is a disciplined way of helping people understand their conditions, situations, and prospects by helping them (at times, unfortunately, insisting that they) grapple with their own moral beliefs, what they really and truly want and believe is worthwhile. The same is true regarding the providers, who have personal beliefs as well but who also practice in professions that make claims on them, embody commitments, and require compliance. You try to help them articulate that sense of worth, working with it within the constraints imposed by the sick person's condition and hopes; and then you do your best to help families and doctors and nurses and others appreciate and respect that.

The clinical ethicist works within this nest of relationships— which sometimes fairly bristle with thorny contention—among people in specific places and circumstances and within the context of rules, policies, laws, and protocols hopefully to achieve some coherence to lives that threaten to shatter in ways that may be quite unexpected. The clinical ethicist is a provoker of talk, of conversations and communication about issues at once humdrum and incredibly sensitive, commonplace and vitally intimate, so that people can understand one another and themselves; so that they can, in the shorthand lingo of the clinic, effectively manage each case.

When sick people are well managed, are actually taken care of in sensitive and intelligent ways, they have much for which to be grateful. Indeed, trying to find appropriate ways to express gratitude is among the most interesting features of the experience of illness. At the same time, we quickly come to realize that doctors have much to be grateful for as well. After all, they are helped to learn and understand—certainly one of the driving motives for becoming a doctor—by sick people. They begin learning on cadavers and pieces of human bodies, sometimes very tiny pieces like cells and fibers. They continue learning by taking our histories and doing physical exams. Eventually they become good clinicians, if they ever do succeed in that difficult art, by learning to elicit important information from us and from our bodies. Patients are decisive for becoming and remaining a doctor.

Recently, it has been urged that we think of ethicists as "facilitators," which is perfectly true, but by itself hardly enough. For what does the ethicist facilitate or enable? And how is this done? With whom? In the course of the stories that follow, my hope is that those sorts of questions will become clearer. At the end of the stories, I expect to address these questions more directly. I also want to tackle what seem to me some of the most pressing and difficult questions an ethics for the twentieth-first century must confront, and thus must be prepared to understand and contend with, hopefully doing so with far greater insight and preparedness than most of us showed in dealing with the harsh issues that have dogged our collective—at times individual—lives over the past few decades. It is probably no exaggeration to say, as have several politicians, that our technological development in this period has far outstripped our moral development. It is a time when the potency of organ transplanting, mechanical ventilators, cardiac surgery, anesthesia, drugs, the new genetics, and the rest of the all-too-familiar catalog of technological goodies has been foisted on us, and we have perhaps been too quick to accept.

All these matters harbor important ethical problems and puzzles. But because my work has been mainly within acute, tertiary-care, regional referral centers, I have been involved in situations that are less embracing and more individual, concerned with the questions faced by acutely ill people. This focus, however, is typical of medicine in our times, and we are only just learning to grapple with the challenges posed by those who are chronically ill. Those challenges, and the harsh problems our society currently faces as attempts are made to recast our health-care system as whole, are not directly part of these narratives. I have no doubts that learning to deal with the ethical issues posed by chronic illness must surely be a main item on any agenda for the future. Moreover, I certainly agree that reforming the system itself—what national priorities and policies should be adopted—is immensely important. On the other hand, that effort should never ignore the fact that health care and illness, acute or chronic, always wear a very personal face.

Policymakers have much to learn from individuals like those in these narratives. But such reflections get me ahead of myself, for making sense of such matters as those really does require a deep appreciation of the difficulties faced by these individuals—which is perhaps best done by going with me through my own early, very puzzled gropings to discover whether and how ethics has a place in these actual clinical situations. I invite you to listen to these stories of people on the edge, to their troubled voices as they try earnestly, and at times desperately, to make sense of themselves, their lives, their futures.

# The Many Ways of Ethics

Trying to do the really right thing can be very difficult. It requires a level of seriousness, measured by many as "objectivity," as being a sort of distance from a situation, something that doesn't come easily. What's more, if we're trying at the same time to be ourselves, to get in touch with our own true feelings, convictions, and values, this distance-seeking is not only awkward but seems oftentimes self-defeating.

Yet it was just this attempt at attaining that objectivity otherwise so often praised that was my first mistake, though hardly my last, as I began over ten years ago to venture (my first true adventure, I should say) through the corridors and wards where physicians and nurses work with patients: the world of clinical medicine. I most definitely was not in any sense a "moralist"; that preoccupation smacks of more confidence in moral affairs than I could muster. Nor was I trying to be an "ethicist," a job as awkward to do as the name is difficult to pronounce. I was hardly ready for any of that, for I hadn't even heard the word "ethicist" at the time I began this perilous adventure. Even less could I understand what a person such as myself was doing there in the hospital, inside clinical wards and units or merely walking the hallways. I was neither sick nor visiting a friend or relative.

But there I was, standing at the battery of monitors at the nurse's station in the cardiac Critical Care Unit (CCU) alongside a couple of residents (I think one of them was an intern, although at the time I didn't appreciate the difference), some medical students, and, of course, the attending physician (I ought to write that in caps: ATTENDING, for that is where the real power and prestige is, as even I in my neophyte stage could tell). All of us were white-smocked and bedecked with the neat blue badge of identified, legitimated admission to these scenes. Mine read, in bold letters:

RICHARD M. ZANER, PH.D.
MEDICAL ETHICS
DEPARTMENT OF MEDICINE

The attending physician, a marvelously gentle human being whose practice was cardiology, led a brief review of each of the patients hooked up to the monitors, asking the residents and students about the status, current therapies, and tests. After the review, the idea was then to go in turn into each room and meet, talk with, and examine each patient. I found myself with the others in a young woman's room. She was hospitalized to undergo a battery of tests to determine whether or not the artificial heart valve implanted several years previously was now failing and might have to be replaced with another. Just thirty-two, she had suffered heart problems since childhood, married when she was twenty-two, had one child when she was twenty-four (under the cautious eye of both obstetrician and cardiologist), and had several valve implants, one at age nineteen and another when she was twenty-seven, the one which now seemed to be failing.

Cheerful, optimistic, and rather attractive, her responses to the attending's questions were articulate, to the point, and clearly showed her to be intelligent and sensitive and have a dry and slightly ironic sense of humor. Since things were very serious for her, I couldn't help but wonder how she could find anything humorous. After further talk, the attending proceeded to pull down the sheet, lift up her gown, and, stethoscope in hand, listen to her heart—first here, then there, then around the side, the back, and again around to the front.

"What the hell am I doing here?" raced through my mind as I stood there stunned, observing what seemed to me such privacies, such intimacies I had no business witnessing. The attending stepped aside to allow the resident to listen to the woman's heart. The intern and each of the students followed suit. This is a teaching hospital, after all, and students must learn to listen and hear such things as failing heart valves. All this time, that inward, whispering voice kept up its insistent challenge: "what am I doing here?" The attending then turned to me—ice sharded down my spine, through my belly, and up again to lodge hard and glaringly obvious in my throat—and asked if I wanted to check out the heart sounds. Before I could really gain any balance sufficient to decline, he handed me his stethoscope and stepped back. The woman, looking utterly unconcerned ("My god," I thought, "doctors really do unhesitatingly break with expected boundaries between people, and with impunity!"), looked up at me as if I, too, were a real doctor and was therefore going to do what any other would do, or had just done. I couldn't just say, "wait a minute, I'm not a real doctor, you see, but only a philosopher, and even though . . ." so I just took the stethoscope (never having used one of the things before), and with my left hand lifted up her left breast a bit (that's what the attending had done), placed the end of the instrument, and plugged the ends into my ears, and listened, moving it a bit to the left side, to the back, around to the right side and front and wondering what the resident, intern, and students must be thinking: "What the hell is he doing there? He's not a real doctor!" I heard a slight thump-de-bump-de-de-whump. I was struck, amazed, so wholly absorbed that I actually forgot where I was; my hands moved on this woman's bare body, touching breast, side, back, listening and hearing. The heart valve could be heard, and what I heard would not have been heard if the valve were functioning correctly.

After we left her room, I let the attending know that I did not appreciate the way he had introduced me, that patients have the right to know who I am and what my position is, and that I would certainly feel more comfortable not to be mistaken for a medical doctor. He quickly agreed and apologized, and we proceeded on to other patients' rooms—without, happily, a repeat of the first encounter.

Later that evening, my wife and I had supper at the cardiologist's home. When we arrived, he took me aside and asked me whether I was insured. Insured in what sense? I had life, home, auto, and accident insurance. Did he mean that? Hardly, I thought. So, in fine form and feeling good that I had survived the morning's encounter without any untoward incident, I said, "Insurance? Hey, George, you think I might be among the first to be sued for moral malpractice?" I chuckled merrily.

He didn't laugh with me. In fact, he looked grave and not a little concerned. "I really need to know, Dick," he said, "because I've written your name in the charts of several patients, and, you realize, patient charts are accessible by courts when there is a legal suit."

"What?" I burbled. "You mean I could be sued?"

"Well, it will doubtless not come to that in this case, of course, but just in case it should happen, now or later, you will certainly have to have insurance, since you could be a party in the suit."

Up bubbled all sorts of horrible images: me standing there with my philosophy hanging out in public, the judge (stern demeanor, of course), the jury (puzzled at this curious "professional," this "expert," standing before them), the prosecuting attorney (looking gleefully at my sweaty face, knowing what a stupid jerk I must be and how his case would now be so easy to win), and a zillion-bucks award being stripped from me (from my very skin, as I couldn't tell you what a million, much less a zillion, bucks even looks like or how long it would take a regular citizen to count, much less to spend such a sum).

And then, as if that were not enough, George asked me what I charge for consults. Charge? For consults? What the hell are those? And, what could "charge" mean for me, a philosopher, an academic, a teacher, not a businessman?

My bewildered look must have told him all he wanted to know, for he said, "You know, like a psychiatrist might charge, or a neurologist if I had to have his expertise in a particular case." Expertise? I'm an expert? In what? Ethics? Is anybody an expert in ethics? Good heavens, what would my philosophy colleagues think of that? They had already had quite a bit of fun with me when, at a general faculty meeting, I had worn my white doctor's coat. I had managed, not for the first time, to spill coffee on my suit coat and, to be presentable at the meeting (it was easy to realize that coats and ties were required attire in the medical school) I had quickly donned the white coat, set off to the meeting, and found myself the butt of a number of joking remarks from my humanities colleagues. So, what could I say? I said the obvious: "I haven't the foggiest, George."

"Well," he replied, "you'd better check it out, as you'll be called on for consults quite often; I found your comments this morning really helpful, and have told others about it. I'm sure they'll be calling on you, too."

Helpful? How in the world had I been I helpful, I wondered. What had I done that was helpful? If I could have just figured that out, maybe I could have begun thinking straight about the other questions George had raised, such as whether or not I needed liability insurance. It was clear to me that it made no sense to think of such matters as consults or insurance unless one was not only helpful but also accountable. But how could I be held accountable? By whom and for what? Philosophers, I suppose, are in some sense accountable— to students, to colleagues, to the profession, to the university. Not only are such things rarely discussed, but "being accountable" here, in the hospital, with patients and families, is an entirely different thing. I know that there have been a few students, out of millions, who have tried to sue universities, departments, even faculty; but those could hardly be compared with what I now seemed to be facing.

In a litigious society like ours, legal suits are far more likely to occur and are likely to be far more damaging, especially regarding health care and physicians, and unlike anything I might even remotely face as a simple professor of philosophy. While I could make some sense of "being helpful" when it comes to students, colleagues, departments, or universities, "being helpful" here with physicians and patients is very different.

I just couldn't make much sense of insurance or consults. So the very next morning, I went to see the chairman of my department (Medicine), urgency fairly plastered all over my face. When I asked about insurance in my case, he, like myself the night before, immediately chuckled: "You mean that you're concerned you might be sued for moral malpractice?" I didn't chuckle, but straight away told him of George's comments, where I had been the day before, what I had observed and done, what I had said, and that George had written me into several charts as having consulted on the cases. As I had done the night before, he quickly shifted gears and advised me to check with someone in Medical School Administration immediately, as he didn't have the slightest idea what to make of the notion of insurance. As for a consultant's fee, he also drew a complete blank, advising me to see the dean about that.

A quick check by the associate vice chancellor for the hospital fortunately showed that, because of the way I was listed on the faculty of the department—Professor of Medicine (Ann Geddes Stahlman Professor of Medical Ethics; philosophy)—I was automatically insured for malpractice. But, I kept thinking again and again, insured against what? What could a legal suit that included me as the consulting ethicist possibly look like? Philosophy has for so long been thought to be so utterly remote from, if not irrelevant to, the real world—the nitty-gritty, push-and-shove world of business, commerce, courts, and such practical things—that being sued in relation to my being a philosopher was a really curious notion. But I wasn't simply a philosopher; whatever else I thought that I was doing in that hospital, my name was being written into patient charts, thus exposing me, like the "real" doctors, to that push-and-shove reality of clinical practice.

Even if insured, even if the idea of suing a philosopher, seemed so odd, it suddenly hit me that, crazy or not, this had become very real, this was something with which I would have to reckon continuously in everything I did from then on. Although I had been cautious and hadn't even picked up, much less looked at or read, any patient chart (I didn't think it was my business, and surely no patient could have possibly bargained on someone like me looking at the chart and all the intimate things it contained), now I would have to be really, truly cautious. And this was only the beginning of how cautious I felt I would have to become. I could never forget my odd position, could never take it for granted, my very presence in the hospital least of all.

As I said, I had begun all this by trying to be objective, serious. This was my first mistake. I had begun that rounding session with the overt expression and demeanor of one who seemed quite serious, even knowledgeable, about things. Surely, though the thought never actually occurred to me that way, patients and doctors and nurses and all the others in the hospital, expect one to be serious. What never occurred to me before all of that was whether I really had anything to be serious about in the first place!

When the scary part happened—at the bedside, touching that woman, pretending to be a doctor, and then that evening when George hit me with the insurance and consult fee bit—there was an exclamation point bubbling about my head complete with comic strip arrows pointing to me: now there is something to be serious about! My own uncovered rearward parts were utterly exposed, and I was left with little more than the awful question about my own accountability. I began to sympathize with the joking (and not-so-joking) references you hear about physicians trying to "cover" those anatomical parts.

The trouble was that while doctors quite literally have some pretty clear and direct things to be worried about, did I? If, as is often said, physicians are there "in the trenches," where was I? If I were to be so exposed, it seemed reasonable, even necessary, that there be some good reason for holding me accountable for something I might do to, with, or on behalf of patients (not to mention for doctors, nurses, and others). Otherwise, I might simply be regarded as a sort of busybody poking around where I didn't belong. How could I be held accountable and even subject to liability? What could I be held accountable for? And to whom?

I must say, that for all the truly frightening aspects of the experience, I learned some things that seemed at once interesting and even important. For example, you really can know with your ears. For centuries, philosophers and psychologists have talked little about that. Instead, they emphasized the eyes, vision. Indeed, traditional definitions of knowledge have not very often taken into account much about hearing, auscultation, or about touching with a knowing focus and purpose, palpation. Much less have these senses, these "data collectors," been taken into account within the theory of knowledge, epistemology. Learning about some of the inner gurglings and burblings of the human body through hearing (amplified, or at least focally aided, by the stethoscope) and touching was a revelation.

I also learned, first hand and with much apprehension, the literal truth of what physician Eric Cassell pointed out regarding the doctor's relation to patients:

> *I remember a patient lying undressed on the examining table, who said quizzically, "Why am I letting you touch me?" It is a very reasonable question. She was a patient new to me, a stranger, and fifteen minutes after our meeting, I was poking at her breasts! Similarly, I have access to the homes and darkest secrets of people who are virtual strangers. In other words, the usual boundaries of a person, both physical and emotional, are crossed with impunity by physicians.*[1]

The relationship between physicians and patients is "a very odd kind of relation between people," Cassell says. And there I was, actually living in and with that odd relation. Who was I for that woman? A doctor? I don't know, frankly, but I do now know, with striking directness, intimacy, and exposure, about the way doctors cross the usual social and moral barriers between people with "impunity."

I also learned something about distance: however intimate I in fact was with that woman's body, I was not an intimate of hers nor she of mine. Intimate was just not the same thing it is when really intimate people get together. I am intimate with my wife and close to my children and to my parents. Like the rest of us, I am also intimate with friends—we talk about things only we know about and know personal things about each other that are no one else's business, for instance. I was not at all intimate with that woman in any of these ways. I didn't "feel" her breasts, did not "caress" her sides or back. I was listening to her heart sounds. Never mind that I was not a medical doctor, for even if I were merely being made to play at being a doctor, there was a tangible sense of distance between us. It was a distance made all the more obvious by what in other respects could only be called intimate actions of touching and listening to her heart sounds.

There is a very fine line here, one that's very easy to collapse— by me certainly, but also by doctors. Even patients can cross it, as I've had to learn. I've come to realize that there are people who act seductively with doctors, patients who forget or get confused about the subtle difference between intimacy and distance. I know that it is very hard to be fully aware of that difference, what with all the touching, looking, listening, talking, and the rest that goes on while first meeting a patient, much less doing a physical examination. It is so difficult that even doctors may also cross that significant line in their relations with patients. The doctor who forgets what he or she is as a doctor and crosses from medically focused examination to intimacy surely violates a crucial barrier that legitimates being a doctor, that authorizes physical examinations and history taking, where through conversation other types of barriers are crossed as well.

Maybe that's why ancient physicians, those early Hippocratic healers, or would-be healers, made such a big deal about this peculiar kind of distance-within-intimacy, or intimacy-within-distance. They worried, for instance, about what could possibly warrant the necessary trust every patient had to have, indeed had no choice but to place, in doctors: trust in their skills, their knowledge, their integrity, even in them as persons. Maybe that's why those ancient physicians so often and pointedly emphasized that the would-be healer must never have sexual relations with patients (or members of their families or households), must always act on behalf of the patient's interests, and must never speak about what is learned in the course of helping a patient. Maybe that's why, too, they placed so much emphasis on the moral virtues of justice and self-restraint. The physician, they believed, must never be unjust or mischievous toward their patients (families, households); nor, they fervently believed, must they allow their patients to do mischief to themselves. The bottom line here, one that was understood to be among the most basic of moral injunctions for physicians, is that the healer must never take advantage of the multiply disadvantaged patient. They realized that to be sick is to be disadvantaged and compromised both by the illness and by the relationship to the doctor, who has the edge over the patient in knowledge, skills, resources, and social legitimation and authority. That fine line I experienced while listening to this patient's heart was a patent, unbreakable moral bond with her, a pact silently but emphatically made by the very action itself—never mind that I was not a "real" doctor. Here, "intimacy" is not intimacy at all; rather, it is a form of distance without which there can be no therapy, no medical help.

"Distance" was taking on new meaning for me, and so was the "seriousness" of my work. For all my embarrassment and bewilderment about accountability—not only concerning the matter of insurance, but more importantly my responsibility to her and to the doctors in the room with me not to take advantage of her vulnerability—I was learning something I had not realized before. Not only did I have to think very hard about so many things for the first time in my life, really, but everything I did or did not do had to be done or not done responsibly. If I said or did anything at all, it couldn't be idly or loosely tossed off; I had to be able to say why I said it (or, say why I did not say something, or anything at all), and this "why" had to be explained and made understandable to others, especially to her.

Even more, I had to keep myself constantly open to criticisms and questions, especially from her. I had to act responsibly in both senses of that marvelously rich idea: at once responsive to whatever concerns she and others voiced and responsible to the people who voiced the concerns; responsive to the specific problems of each case and responsible for everything I said and did. Whatever else the idea of accountability could mean for someone like me in these settings, nothing could be taken for granted as obvious, for myself most of all.

Trying to do good things for people can be awfully difficult when you are serious, especially when you don't know what "being serious" amounts to. Maybe some part of that distance-within-intimacy or intimacy-within-distance, so vividly present to me while I listened to that woman, has to do with learning what seriousness is all about: that fine line that is at once so tangible in actual practice but so difficult to talk about when removed from those encounters.

# T W O

# There's Always a First Time

Rounds with my cardiologist friend was only part of my early experiences. I was also actively involved with the daily rounds of the Newborn Intensive Care Unit (NICU) and with Hematology-Oncology, to name a couple. Each of them had its own style, customs, and rituals that also needed to be learned and respected; individualism is very much at home in the world of clinical practice. The hematologists, along with their team of residents, interns, students, nurses, and social worker, went from one room to another seeing and talking with each patient, while other teams would merely meet outside each patient's room and discuss their current statuses, only rarely going into the room.

The NICU is a different thing altogether. It included several large rooms, two with space for twelve seriously ill babies each and a third room with space for approximately six babies needing intermediate care. There was also one small isolation room that could accommodate about four babies with contagious diseases. At that time the unit could handle as many as thirty-four or thirty-five babies; the space and number of beds has since increased. There was one primary-care nurse for each baby; as many as two or three residents in their second or third year of clinical training in pediatrics, each of whom had some supervisory role; usually four or five interns in their first year of training, each of whom was responsible for providing primary care for four to six babies; one fellow in neonatology responsible for supervising the residents and interns and, at times, serving as attending physician; and one attending physician responsible for all treatment decisions in the unit. (Each of four attendings rotated on a monthly basis; when not serving as attending, the others were typically engaged in research.) So, rounding each morning in the NICU were residents and interns rotating in different units of pediatrics on different schedules, several nurses, the Fellow, and the attending.

When I first arrived at the medical center, the NICU was one of the first units I started to visit. Of course, shortly after I accepted my position, the "Baby Doe" issue began to heat up, giving a rather more substantial reason for including me in discussions. By the time the avid public disputes began in early 1982, I already had some experience with the kinds of problems these professionals regularly faced. At the beginning, however, I was dumbfounded by the sheer presence of all that equipment and those technological devices with their buzzers and lights and the dots and blips and lines on monitor screens; the hushed, fervent activity of nurses and doctors bending over the babies' beds; the beds and isolets in turn hung with name-cards, some with ribbons and pictures, some with scrawled greetings from parents and families, some with nothing; and the babies. Most of the babies were "preemies," little more than a handful in size, whose ages at birth could be read from the cards: 34 weeks, 36 weeks, 30 weeks. There on that bed in the middle of the room, no bigger than a kitten, was a baby with a gestational age of 25 weeks. Tiny, wrinkled-skinned, and gnarled-looking; plugged into monitors, intubated, and connected to mechanical ventilators; lights mounted on cribs to maintain temperature, feeding tubes looped and coiled with fluids and medicines and proteins, other tubes for tapping the blood supply to keep checks on electrolytes and minerals—all worked in an incredibly complex delicate balancing act to keep this girl, that boy, those twins, alive and "intact" neurologically.

In one place, another team of physicians were riveted in focused attention as a surgeon, masked, with magnifier glasses in place, tracked the incredibly precise and minute maneuvers of his hands as they gently carved and pierced and levered into one small body. In another place, a technician, having wheeled in an elephant-sized machine to hover over another slight figure, whirred it into photometric action. And everywhere the gentle clunks and wheezes and zaps of ventilators kept airways open, pushed oxygen into small and undeveloped lungs, some doing this with greater force and faster pace than others. Everything in the NICU, or most everything, was designed simply to do for the babies what their more natural places in their mothers' wombs do far better.

Standing next to the nurses and doctors on rounds discussing the problems, tests, diagnoses, medications, and nutrition for each baby in turn and listening to them only gave me further reason for being stunned: none of it made any sense, neither technical terms nor numbers nor percentages nor problems nor diagnoses. None of it sounded familiar, rang any bells, or set off light bulbs of understanding in me. If not technical terms and numbers, they seemed wont to talk initials. And I was too embarrassed, or at the moment too compacted with urgency, to ask what even some of it might mean. Once I heard "PTA" and wondered what that could mean; I later found out, thanks to a nurse who took pity on me, that it stood for "prior to admission." That left me wondering dizzily if everything had to be said with initials? Even that? Then I heard "PDA" and, thinking of so much that seemed, in my naiveté, trivial yet pronounced with real gravity, I thought here it goes again! Only to find out that this set of initials carried awesome weight. "Patent ductus arteriosus," a resident said, which, I learned, can be literally life threatening: the path of blood circulation of the fetus bypasses the lungs through this duct, since it does not need its blood oxygenated but gets this through the mother, but if that duct doesn't close after birth (which it normally does, but is a frequent issue for preemies), it could mean death for the baby because blood isn't properly oxygenated, a potential disaster.

So from baby to baby I trailed behind baffled and straining to
hear what was said, not wanting to interrupt what was an obviously
important set of discussions that left little time for my anxious
questions and trying to take notes so that, later, I could look up a few
things I could later ask about and begin to understand. Sometimes
an attending would stop, look up, focus, and pounce on me:

**Attending:** We've been beating on this baby now for two
months, doing everything we know how, but she's just not
responding at all well, and if we keep this up and she manages
to be a survivor she likely won't be intact; she may well die
before she reaches her fourth birthday; or, if she does survive,
she'll likely be physically debilitated and mentally retarded,
probably quite severely. Should we keep it up?

**Me (to myself):** "Beating"? "Not responding"? "A survivor"?
"Intact"? "Debilitated"? "Retarded"? How the hell would I
know what to do? I don't even know what in the world he
means by all these words much less what "doing everything"
means or what it takes to help this baby "do well." Why ask
me?

**Me (aloud):** I'm not sure what you mean by "being an intact
survivor." Thus, I'm not sure what you are asking me.

**Me (to myself):** Brilliant, Zaner. There's a real answer for you.
Time to get out of here, for sure.

**Attending:** Well, she just can't take these ventilator settings,
and we can't get them down any further, we can't wean her
down, and if we keep them up her lungs can't take it and will
start to die; what we're doing to help will soon start to kill her.
Yet, if we don't keep it up, she'll die for lack of ability to
breath properly. Either way, we're on a course that can't seem
to be changed. What do you think we should do?

**Me (to myself):** Good lord, what's helping is also hurting, yet
if they stop that'll kill her, too. What to do? How do I know?

**Me (aloud):** What do her parents think? Do they understand what's going on? They may not want you to continue, if they think it's hopeless, that what you're doing is causing more harm than benefit; they may not really understand what's going on. In any case, they can't be expected to give their informed consent if they don't understand, and you can't expect to continue treating the baby if what you're doing is no benefit, is in effect causing more harm than doing good.

**Attending:** Good question! Well, Bob [the resident], have you talked with them recently? I haven't had the chance to meet with them yet. Who's talked with them?

And so it went for the first few months I was there: them asking me horrendous, awesome questions presumably—actually—expecting something helpful in response; me fumbling, fidgeting, mumbling, and eventually (if I was lucky) coming up with something modestly pertinent.

That I gradually got used to things goes, I suppose, without saying. But getting used to things and having a sense that you actually belong there, are not the same experience! The Baby Doe dispute was in full swing, with nationwide publicity being given to the case back East. She was a little girl born with spina bifida (the spinal cord protruded from a lesion and she had developed hydrocephalus as a result) and microcephaly (abnormally small head and brain). The prognosis for survival for this tiny baby was extremely poor, and even if she did survive, with all the NICU help that could be mustered on her behalf, she would in all likelihood have grave physical problems and serious mental retardation. Her parents had thus decided, with religious advice and support, not to have her treated. The physicians and hospital concurred. Somehow, a self-described "right-to-life" attorney heard of the case and sued to force the surgery. The case then went through each of that state's courts, eventually winding up as a national news story. Finally, with that state's highest court concurring with the parents' decision, it was appealed to the U.S. Supreme Court, which ruled in favor of the parents. The case was based on the federal government's interpretation of Section 504 of the Rehabilitation Act of 1973, which, the Court stated, did not give authority to gain access to the baby's medical records without parental permission. The government's efforts were declared unconstitutional.

One day I was telephoned at my office and asked for urgent help. While I had been fairly well accepted in the NICU and had even apparently been of some help in several cases, I had never had such a call. "Urgent?" I asked. The response chilled me: yes, there was an urgent problem, and the attending had asked me if I would help. So, I went careening down the hallways of the office building, heart pounding, nerves atingle, and ran head-on into the hospital chaplain. "Hey, Zaner," he shot after me as I kept on running, "got an urgent call?" "I guess so," I replied and then stopped in my tracks, stunned at my audacity, thinking that the attending may have a screw loose somewhere. Help? Me? I wondered to myself, as I started up again on my way to the hospital. How?

Getting to the NICU, I learned that a young couple's first babies, twins, were not only extremely premature at birth (25 weeks, as I recall), but also that each was born with serious congenital anomalies. Neither was expected to make it, although one looked a bit better than the other. "The trouble is," the attending told me, "we can't get the parents to understand the situation. The mother does talk some, but the father hasn't said a word." The problem, as the attending saw it, was the father. Several efforts to communicate with him seemed to have failed; he just didn't talk, though he appeared to be listening, and it was unclear whether he really understood what was being said about his babies. More than that, it was known that both he and his wife were college graduates and that the father had some sort of executive position in a local corporation. The worry, as it came out, was that the father, clearly intelligent, might be thinking about a legal suit to force treatment, an action, physicians and nurses agreed, that would not be appropriate for either twin. "See if you can find out what's going on with him," he told me, "we need to know, for at least one twin is going to die regardless of what we are doing, and the other, too, most likely."

In this NICU, the preferred decision-making model was to have key decisions shared. The attending would give his or her best medical judgment along with a recommended course of action; then the parent(s) would either agree or not, as the case may be. At this time, moreover, the place of parents as decision makers was under severe scrutiny by the Federal government's Department of Health and Human Affairs (DHHS), itself under pressure from several child-advocacy groups. Hence, not only was there much public pressure to keep treating, but also considerable caution about parents making such life-and-death decisions. This case, then, was viewed as especially difficult on both counts.

I set up a meeting with the parents. When they arrived, we went into a quiet room. Not having done this before, I wasn't at all sure just what should be done, much less by someone like me. Moreover, it was unclear to me just what these parents expected when they were asked to talk with me, an ethicist. What did most of us think, especially a decade ago, about having "an ethics discussion"? Probably that something was really wrong, that someone had erred or done something very inappropriate. Otherwise, why talk to an ethicist? Moreover, I knew full well how much publicity had been generated by the Baby Doe disputes, so it seemed reasonable to expect them to know about it and probably to have some questions about the ethics of handling their babies.

I was both right and wrong. Right, they knew a good deal about the Baby Doe issues; but wrong, oh so wrong, about what I thought might be on their minds, the father especially. He had seen one of the "Nightline" shows several weeks prior. It was devoted to the Baby Jane Doe affair and included such details as the father of that girl testifying in one of the courts with a paper bag over his head in order, he said, "to protect what remains of my privacy!" That had impressed the father in my case, so much so that he thought he had the matter all figured out. He fully understood what the physicians and nurses had been telling him and, even in his grief and anxiety, was perfectly clear about what should, in his mind, be done: withdrawal of life supports was, he said, "the only humane thing to do," as everything currently being done was "merely prolonging dying, and that is just wrong!" When I asked why he hadn't been saying this to the staff, as they had been deeply puzzled over his silence, he replied that if he made them make the decision to withdraw supports by keeping his silence, then any legal consequences and publicity would fall on them, not on him and his wife. He desperately wanted to protect his wife and both their families from anything like what that Baby Jane Doe father had been put through.

Resolving the matter then turned out to be surprisingly easy: for his babies' sakes, he needed to communicate with the staff, let them know what and how he felt and especially let them know that he agreed with their recommendation to withdraw life supports as treatments were futile (a criterion for withdrawal that later became part of the Federal law). He had little idea that he had only been making matters worse, since the physician was not about to withdraw treatment without the parents' understanding and agreement. He was in effect responsible for what he himself believed was "inhumane" prolonging of the dying process.

Part of this case, as it turned out, concerned his and his wife's reluctance to put doctors and nurses on the spot by actually request-ing withdrawal of treatments. They were afraid they would be regarded as "bad parents," a term they had overheard being used about another set of parents. They also were reluctant, as are many patients and families, even to appear to put the physician on the spot. They understood that they were in his debt and that of the nurses, that they were very busy with all the other babies in the NICU and were reluctant to "bother" them.

On the other hand, they felt free to talk about all sorts of things with me. "You're not a doctor," his wife said, meaning, among other things, that I had the time to listen to them. And, though they were initially a bit leery about talking to "someone in ethics who, you know, might be judgmental," they quickly responded to assurances that I was not there to judge them or the doctors. In fact, both of them became very intrigued with the fact that I was actually on the scene and able to see them and help them express what was most worthwhile, their "ethics," that is—their feelings, hopes, frustrations. I recall telling him at one point: "you know, you haven't avoided making a decision by your silence; rather, you've merely decided to keep your silence and let others decide—which, you must realize, is itself quite a significant decision."

I have thought a lot about this case ("re-flected upon" is the more proper term, I suppose, though "bounced off" better describes my experience) and have had much to wonder about. As one NICU attending put it to me, "What do you do that any good friend, or even nice, sensitive person, couldn't do?" What, indeed? Certainly, it was no part of my own education or training as a philosopher to get into these sorts of conversations with other people. Nor does being a philosopher equip one to be especially perceptive about these awesomely sensitive dimensions of every person's life, the "what's worthwhile," as I've come to call that realm of feelings, beliefs, urges, and values we call our morality. Sure, we talk endlessly about "ethics" and whatever may be regarded as embraced by that topic. Opinions on that vary from philosopher to philosopher, even from time to time, perhaps. But we philosophers have had nothing like clinical training.

So, the attending's question was not in the least out of court; it hit directly on one of the many matters I'd been running into and had not been able to resolve for myself. First, was I any different from any good friend? Second, even if there was something distinctive about my being a philosopher, just what was that? In short form, the ultimate question gaped before my startled eyes: What in the world is a philosopher doing in the hospital? Is there a legitimate place for a philosopher in clinical settings? What might that be? What, if anything, in my education and training could aid and abet that clinical involvement? If nothing, should there be?

I like to think, of course, that the help provided to those parents and hospital staff was genuine and stemmed from my profession itself: it was as a philosopher that I helped, I hope. I am quite a bit clearer about all that today, certainly much more so than I was then, for all I could do in the face of that attending's question was mumble. But the issue bedeviled my tracks for years; it wouldn't let go, and

I couldn't ignore it even if I tried. Physicians and nurses kept me reminded of it, and also I'm reminded of an encounter twenty years ago when I was really a neophyte at this business.

It occurred during my first year in this field at the State University of New York at Stony Brook. After accepting the appointment to the medical school, I was being introduced to the school's executive committee on which, as director of the Division of Social Sciences and Humanities in Medicine, I would soon begin to serve. I had already learned, during my interviews there, that it was deadly to introduce me as a "philosopher," for that introduction was regularly greeted with stunned silence, and apparently the acting dean had also learned not to do this. When he got up to do the introducing, he said to the assembled heads of departments and divisions, "This is Dr. Zaner, he's our resident phenomenologist." That's my philosophical specialty, one could say, but I had assiduously avoided using the term for fear it would create even more confusion than "philosopher." To my amazement, things went swimmingly, no curious looks, no raised eyebrows, no behind-the-hand smirks.

Puzzling about this, I thought I'd figured it out. There is neurology, physiology, biology, pathology, and . . . phenomenology. They must think I've got a medical specialty, I thought. I was wrong. The acting dean, when I asked him what he understood by "phenomenology," said, "well, you're our communications expert, aren't you?" Communications? I wondered how in the world he ever got that idea, but I kept my silence and let it pass. Only years later did it occur to me that he could be right, though he might not have realized just how right he was. Beyond the conundrum lies something of an insight: philosophers do have the misfortune to be in love with ideas, with the language by which we express our ideas. I suppose, then, that being a philosopher, more especially being a phenomenologist, means that I am deeply concerned with language, with words, with conversations, and with the effort to figure out what we mean by our words— and, in the case of clinical medicine, with those sensitive, often compressed conversations that occur at every bedside. The trick is to try and reflect on those conversations in a way that few of us typically do. We must consider them as we consider our own most basic sense of what's worthwhile in situations that are frequently urgent and demanding and that call for as much clarity and understanding as can be mustered in the circumstances. So the idea that a clinical ethicist focuses on language, on conversations among people, is very much on target, and I've come to appreciate over the years being introduced both as a clinical ethicist and as a phenomenologist.

# THREE

# Iced Beer and Old Friends

Many years later, most of the ethical issues occasioned by acute illness became much clearer and many thorny questions fairly well resolved. So much so that I felt comfortable proposing a clinical ethics program for a local hospital. I was actually contacted by the head of their ethics committee to help figure out the best way to provide an ethics consultation service and educational activities for their physicians and nursing staff. It seemed a good idea to do a pilot project and, at the same time, study it carefully, something that had not been done in depth prior to this. After the pilot, we'd all have some better idea of whether or not it was a good thing.

The idea, which actually worked out rather well, was: a six-month pilot, with several of my senior clinical ethics fellows and I sharing responsibilities for selected teaching and clinical settings. We proposed a number of in-services for the nursing staff, rounds for the medical personnel, and consultations with patients, families, physicians, and nurses in the hospital's intensive care units. We also agreed to meet regularly with the pastoral care staff, hold once-a-month ethics grand rounds, and meet with each of the medical and surgical departments. As this was among the first such programs to be provided by a university-based ethics team at a private hospital, and the first to be done by non-physicians,[1] I thought it was imperative that we study it as carefully as possible, and this was headed up by a colleague who was particularly well equipped for this task.

As the majority of physicians at the hospital are in private practice, we did not expect a great deal of enthusiasm at first; we were right, though this changed considerably as our pilot program progressed. Very soon after the program began, the nursing staff brought to our attention a patient who seemed to need clinical ethics attention. One of the ethics fellows saw her first and took down the basic facts of her case.

The patient, Mrs. Oland, was a seventy-year-old woman, the mother of three adult children, who had been married to a wonderfully gentle and caring man for many years. Mr. Oland, his son, and one daughter were regular visitors during the four and a half months she had been hospitalized with prolonged hypotension, recurrent pneumothorax, respiratory failure, and end-stage renal disease. At the time we saw her, she was not very alert or well oriented and could not make decisions for herself; her prognosis was described as "dismal," for she was not expected to recover kidney function nor be weaned from the ventilator. Nevertheless, Mr. Oland, on whom decision making had fallen, was reported to be unable to accept this bad news and wanted "everything possible" done.

After talking with the kidney specialist who shared attending responsibilities with a pulmonologist, it seemed clear that she would never recover sufficiently to be discharged from the hospital, though this was exactly what the family thought they wanted. Knowing how difficult sound and directed conversations are in hospital settings, it seemed to me that their apparently confused hope was certainly a factor here. I thus felt that a special conference was needed bringing together the family, the attendings, the primary-care nurses, the hospital chaplain, and any others directly concerned with her care.

Before that took place, it was clear from talking with Mr. Oland and his daughter Janice that neither they nor the other children really understood what discharge to home would involve. Talking with him and his son about their wanting "everything possible" done, revealed that though they understood the gravity of her condition and even acknowledged that the physicians and nurses had done "everything," they still wanted to feel sure that "everything" really had been done. Discharge to home, were that at all possible, would have meant that they would be directly and immediately taking care of her. Leaving her in the hospital meant that they were leaving things in others' hands. It thus appeared that they were in the throes of a kind of anticipatory guilt and grieving process. They feared that at some future time they would be locked into an unresolvable "what if" or "if only we had thought of . . . then we would have done things differently." A time for the family to be together—for reflecting on things, for reviewing everything—was clearly a prominent need. The idea for the conference thus took on greater urgency. Rather than doing this alone, however, the family wanted to have all the primary caregivers present, a proposal that struck me as right on target. That way the entire situation could be gone over, with options identified and perhaps even decisions reached.

The entire group met the next morning. After a careful review of the medical facts, with family member's questions and concerns aired (especially about the impossibility of home care for this woman), the options were pinpointed. Only two seemed at all reasonable, given the family's values and the woman's medical condition. The treatment could continue as at present, including dialysis, ventilatory support, etc., in which case she would hang on for perhaps six months. But this would occur only if no other problems occurred—infection, other illness, etc. Since that seemed quite unlikely, she would die despite the "everything" that could be done, with her dying and their grieving merely prolonged. On the other hand, the physician could withdraw life supports to allow her to die with as much dignity as was possible in the circumstances, including withdrawal of dialysis or ventilation or both. As everyone wanted her to be as comfortable as possible, provision for palliative care, especially relief from anxiety and pain, was a high priority. It was recommended that dialysis be discontinued first. According to the renal specialist, Mrs. Oland would experience little, if any, pain or discomfort and would gradually lapse into a coma after a few days, and then peacefully die. Since she would at that time become unconscious and no longer experience anxiety or pain, it was decided that it would then be appropriate to withdraw the ventilator, so as not to prolong the inevitable. After much discussion, the family finally agreed that these were the measures that should be taken. They all seemed comfortable with this decision, and steps to implement it were taken.

The conference was marked by unusual candor. Still, it seemed to me that something important was not voiced, so I decided to talk with Mr. Oland again. The next morning I found him in his wife's room and asked him to step outside for a moment. His daughter Janice joined us.

At one point, he said, "Dr. Langston just shouldn't say things like that."

"Like what?" I asked.

"Well," he paused, "you know, that Martha's just doing no good and . . . well . . ."

He seemed unable to go on. Janice and I sat quietly, waiting. Mr. Oland glanced at her, but her eyes, dimmed with grief, were averted.

"It just seems to me," he slowly continued, "that you shouldn't say, just right out like that, that . . . that . . . Martha wouldn't want us to help, to get her better so's we can get her back home." His voice became increasingly assertive. "I know what the doctors and others said in the conference yesterday. But it is just so *unfair*, don't you know? *Home*, that's where she belongs. *That's* where she *belongs*, and where she *wants* to be. *Dammit*, she just don't want to be in this damned hospital. We *got* to get her out of here and back home. Now you listen to me, young man, you got to tell that doctor that Martha's got to be done *right*, taken home, and I just don't care what he says . . ."

Janice seemed stung. She looked up at him, surprised, and murmured, "Oh, Daddy, don't, just don't." Looking at me, she pled, "Please, you've got to understand. Daddy is just so upset, he . . ."

"Janice," Mr. Oland broke in, "just hush, right now. You *know* Mamma don't like this place, don't like it *at all*. You *know* that, and you know we've just *got* to get her back *home* where she belongs. It just ain't *right* to ask us to leave her here, what with all that damned stuff hooked up to her, and her barely breathin' and strugglin' so much. I already talked to her and she told me so."

"You already discussed this with her?" I broke in. "But you haven't mentioned this before. Are you sure?"

"Well . . ." again he was having difficulty getting his thoughts into words. "Well, yeh, in a way. You know, before she began to fade here a month or so ago." He continued rapidly. "But that ain't the point anyway. I just *know* what Martha'd want and not want, and she wants to go *home*."

"I know, Daddy, I know," Janice said, sobbing softly.

The conversation began to flag then, and I thought that we'd done enough for now. In the hallway, after Mr. Oland had returned to his wife's room, Janice drew me aside. "You've got to understand, Dr. Zaner. Daddy is just not himself. All that language, it's just not like him."

"He certainly seems rather disturbed and angry . . ."

"But that's just the point, you see, he's not *angry*, that's just not his way at all. He's such a sweet, gentle man. He *never* uses words like that, never talks to people that way. I *know* something's wrong, that he's really bothered about something; otherwise he wouldn't act that way. I thought we had talked it all out, that he understood, especially after that conference . . . not just that Mamma isn't going to make it, but that we just can't take her home. I *know* he knows."

"What do you think is on his mind, then?"

She went on to say that she felt he was deeply disturbed about something, but when she had talked with him before I had first met with them he seemed increasingly closed up. He wouldn't talk to her, not the way he most often did, and when she asked several times what was bothering him he just clammed up. She thought that in the conference he'd gotten whatever it was under control. He was more like his "real self" then, she emphasized.

"But when we talked after the meeting, well, that's just not like him. We've always been able to talk about the most difficult things. Now . . ." she hesitated, trying to find the words, "now, I just know that something's wrong."

"Don't you think it's important to find out what it is? It's not going to help if he stays angry and upset."

"But, I don't think he's angry, you see?"

"I'm sorry, I didn't mean 'angry,' but he does seem quite upset. What's going on? Do you have any idea?"

"Well, I'm not sure, but I know what you mean, about the importance of finding out and all. There's something festering inside him, and he won't admit it. Can you help?"

"Let me be candid. Are any of you worried about something with the feeding tube? That's something that wasn't addressed very directly in the meeting, and it occurred to me that might be what's bothering your father. You know, the newspapers and TV have been filled with the topic, what with the Cruzan case going on now and the Supreme Court soon to decide the case."

"Feeding tube?" she asked. "What do you mean? Isn't that just one of those life supports that aren't going to be kept up now? Why would we worry about that?"

"You're *not* worried?"

"Not at all."

"But what about your father?"

"No, I don't think so. We all talked about all that yesterday before the conference, and . . . no, I don't think any of us is concerned about that."

"Well, the reason I mention it is that some people seem to think that pulling the feeding tube is the same thing as starving a person. And though, from everything I know, that is not an appropriate concern, it is terribly symbolic . . ."

"We know all that, Dr. Zaner, but, really, that hasn't bothered us."[2]

So much for my suspicion. What, then, was behind his behavior? As Janice and I continued to talk, it seemed to me that there was indeed an underlying issue eating at him. I wasn't sure how to get to it, but another conversation seemed in order. He was willing, so we went back into the conference room. With considerable courage, he was eventually able to dredge it up. He had somehow managed to get it in his mind that *he* was to blame for the crisis that led to his wife being hospitalized. While he knew that she had had "problems" for a long time, she had remained very active. He said he hadn't really tried to persuade her to take it easier, and he felt that he *should* have tried. Yet beneath that increasingly corrosive sense of guilt, there was still something else going on. In a way, he recognized that his sense of guilt over not being more persistent in getting her to ease off just didn't ring true. The oppressive "something else" then gradually came out.

Mrs. Oland had been very aware of her condition for some time and was quite concerned over what was likely to happen if she had to be hospitalized. More than once she had tried to talk about the matter, especially about her death. He softly told me that she had really tried to talk about precisely what in fact had happened, about "all those tubes and things." But he simply *could not* talk about that; it meant he would have to face losing her. Nor could he face the dreadful prospect of sitting day after day in the waiting room, seeing her so infrequently, finding her too debilitated to talk, and, most of all, living without her among the countless things they had shared for so many years. He wasn't angry so much as experiencing profound grief. Coupled with that was a harsh but veiled sense of guilt: *he hadn't allowed her to talk,* especially about what she wanted the doctors to do, nor even about her death. When they had asked him if he knew what she wanted, he was stunned into silence. *He didn't know* because he hadn't wanted her to talk about it; he couldn't face it or bring himself even to think about those awesome matters.

Surprises always happen in life, and this time was no exception. Soon after dialysis was discontinued, Mrs. Oland, strangely enough, began to recover some alertness. Discussions with her that were previously impossible had then become imperative, and she made it quite plain that she did not want to continue with "everything." Indeed, she had apparently been trying to say just that for some time, but being on the ventilator and unable to speak, being too weak to write, and fading in and out of wakefulness made it quite difficult for anyone to know whether she was trying to communicate, much less just what she had wanted to say. Responding to questions through nods and hand gestures, she indicated that she had led a rich and rewarding life and was ready for death; all she really wanted was the chance to be with her whole family one last time.

This was arranged by transferring her to a larger room closer to the stairway, thereby allowing everyone to visit more freely than otherwise. That night, a kind of party took place with the room about as crowded as it could be. Although she had not eaten at all well before this, she did that night, even indulging (through the feeding tube) in a can of frozen beer! Her son told me that everyone was deeply moved, his mother included, by the several days of discussions and deliberations. All that remained, she told him, was for her to see her best friend, who lived far away and was, unfortunately, unable to be there that evening. But, in fact, she did come a couple days later. This last visit apparently meant a good deal to Mrs. Oland, for she managed to stay quite alert for the intervening two days and visit with her friend for several hours. After the visit she seemed at peace with herself and relaxed into a kind of sleep, slipping deeper and deeper into unconsciousness. She died the next morning.

The entire thing went so smoothly, had such a natural feel to it, that I couldn't help but wonder why I'd been called on for help in the first place. What did anything that went on have to do with "ethics"—a question I've grown used to asking myself with embarrassing regularity. Most often when "ethics" gets mentioned, if it ever does, people generally have it in mind that some big deal is about to happen, or has already occurred. Most often, especially in hospital situations, many people think that someone has done something wrong and that it is the ethicist's job to correct it, or something like that. People nowadays seem inevitably to think of ethics as something akin to law: you don't go to court unless something bad has happened, and then it is the court's job to right the wrong as best it can. Or, ethics is thought to be something like religion: the "bad" is a bit like "sin," and the idea seems to be that the ethicist serves our secular times as a kind of substitute for the priest and the confessional. Or, as I've also regularly found, when "ethics" is mentioned many people just lose patience, apparently thinking that each is his or her own ethicist (so goes the individualism of our times) and that nobody in his or her right mind would need a "specialist" in ethics, for that would be to own up to an embarrassing sort of ineptness.

The encounter with this marvelous family might have seemed, at first blush, to call for one or the other of those responses. Yet, no law had been violated. So what did "ethics" have to do with this case? And if there were something legally suspicious, an attorney, not an ethicist, would be in order. If, on the other hand, ethics is indeed religion, then I hardly met the role of even a secular priest. All I did was convene a meeting, moderate it, and then back out to let things take their course. I had been asked to consult by the attending physician. As he told me later, he thought that the family might feel somewhat freer to talk about things with "people like you." When he first talked with me, interestingly, he too felt quite strongly that something still unspoken was troubling this family. In asking me for a consult, he hoped that I might be able to ferret it out. He also reminded me of my own words in an earlier conversation with him when I told him that I often felt rather like a detective, and he proceeded to lay out what he took to be a "clue." When he had mentioned the possibility of a feeding tube, he had noted a kind of strained reaction. The atmosphere markedly changed, and he decided that, as this was not an immediate issue, he would be better off not pursuing the topic just then.

There was indeed something there, though it turned out to be rather different from what he suspected. During our last conversation,

Mr. Oland said that his wife had told him about a friend who had yanked out her feeding tube; she didn't want "the damned thing," did not want her death prolonged. The story jolted him and he immediately recoiled. Locked in grief and guilt, he just couldn't think, much less talk, about that, so it just sat there silently bubbling beneath the surface. Confronted with the need to decide, and faced with the fact of his wife's condition, he was struck dumb. Having to face the prospect that his wife was going to die, and realizing that he soon had to witness it, was monstrous and unutterable. But eventually, he was able to face the issue, and the situation began to clear up.

Eventually, his loving and gentle wife was resolute in her determination to be allowed to die—even more, to rescue her husband from his suffering and what remained of her own sense of dignity. She finally managed to have her voice heard. She understood what was happening to him and her children and grieved especially over her husband's guilt. In the end, she was even able to help all of them accept her death. She went with dignity into that good night despite the family's hope-against-hope of "doing everything" that had initially brought me into their lives.

This encounter happened many years after I had begun to get involved in these sorts of situations and had already learned a good deal about them, enough to know right off that ethical issues are most often deeply buried, rarely recognized as such, and may require a good deal of indirectness to deal with them appropriately. Kierkegaard, that master of irony and the subtleties of human life, knew this best of all, for he knew enough to know that such matters can only be talked about by not talking about them directly. Indirect discourse, in his words, is the only way to go about understanding things human, especially matters of ethics. So, what I had learned to do is never to talk about "ethical issues," or rather to talk about them by never talking about them. What happened in the case of the Olands seems to fit that idea rather well: feeling that something was really bothering him, it seemed to me that the thing to do was just give him a chance to talk, to come to what was wrong in his own way and at his own pace. Even when he began to talk, though, the thing lying deeply buried beneath even his terrible grief still took time to emerge, and then did so only very gradually, as if testing the light of day for any treacherous snares that might be lying about. Not talking about his grief and guilt directly was a way of letting him talk about them indirectly. People faced with such difficult decisions know this well. Such is the irony of human experience communicated.

> Jack can see he sees
> > what he can see Jill can't see
> and he can see
> > that Jill can't see that she can't see
> but he can't see WHY
> > Jill can't see that Jill can't see.

> Jill
> > can see that he does not understand her
> and can see that he can't see that he doesn't:
> and she can see
> > that he can't see that he can't see
> > > she sees he can't see he doesn't.
> Why does she still feel confused?
> She cannot understand why he can't see that
> she sees that he can't see that he does not understand.

Or:

> There must be something the matter with him
> > because he would not be acting as he does
> > > unless there was
> > therefore he is acting as he is
> > because there is something the matter with him.

> He does not think there is anything the matter with him because
> > one of the things that is
> > the matter with him
> > is that he does not think that there is anything
> > the matter with him

therefore
> we have to help him realize that,
> the fact that he does not think there is anything
> the matter with him
> is one of the things that is
> the matter with him.[3]

Talking about human experience is remarkably different from living it. Talking about clinical ethics is remarkably different from engaging it. The need for clinical ethics intervention often begins as a mere hunch—or, more honestly, as a feeling of helplessness on the part of health-care providers. It is not a technical helplessness, but a relational disease that often steers a physician or nurse toward ethical consult—which in situations like this seems more a form of indirect than direct discourse.

I suppose that when confronted with the need to act and faced with the actual "going to die" that haunts the human spirit when faced, unavoidably, with the specter of death, the family, physicians, and nurses were struck dumb—were awed—by the actual prospect. Yet, that gentle, loving woman so courageous and resolute in her determination to rescue what remained for her of human dignity had the "last say." Neither treatments nor feeding, tears nor fruitless wishing could reverse things, could stay the inexorable course of her disease. In the end, she had her way, going gently into that good night and loved by all those involved in caring for her.

# F O U R

# Exorcising Demons

I mentioned that from the first days at the medical center I was able to move freely throughout the hospital observing almost any clinical activity and being invited to participate in many of them. In retrospect, this openness was probably due, at least initially, to my having been appointed to a very prestigious chair in medical ethics. Never mind that few, if any, people actually knew what could be expected of such a person, or why a chair had been established in the field. Fact is, as I liked to tell folks curious about my being there, this was the first academic position I had ever held where I was able to define my own position: whatever I happened to be doing at any time, well, that was what "ethicists" did. Recognizing that this freedom could also be a license to idleness, I tended to go to the opposite extreme: doing far more than I really had time, much less the wits, to do. I had decided before coming to the center that those of us involved in ethics and medicine had better find out whether or not there really were defensible reasons for our presence and whether we could be at all helpful in those settings where medical ethics issues arise in the first place, in clinical situations.

Then I could get on about the task of being an ethicist. I was going on rounds in many units and learning far more and faster than

I could readily absorb. I was also doing some teaching, both in the medical school and in several departments on the main campus. The rounds were especially preoccupying and fascinating to me. I was taken by the terrible sorts of problems that children and babies faced, problems that, I grew to realize, were common in the newborn intensive care unit and in sophisticated pediatric units.

The hospital where I work is a tertiary, extremely high-tech referral center with the most difficult medical problems being matters of routine practice. Being there on the scene and in the midst of things seemed almost surreal, as if I'd found myself suddenly transported into a science fiction odyssey. Underscoring the surrealism even more was the fact that I did not yet have the sense that I truly belonged there or that I had anything pertinent and practical to contribute. For the most part, I merely listened in, nodding wisely (philosophers are hardly worth their mettle if they don't learn to nod wisely) looking sage, observing, and trying to learn. There were, I acknowledge, many days of severe doubt over what I had gotten myself into.

I recall one especially remarkable child, a two-and-a-half-year-old boy. I first saw him in one of the main pediatric units, walking, quite fast. He had tubes running out of his arm and chest and up to the metal, wheeled carrier to the attached bags of fluid. Jabbering loudly at everyone, he adroitly maneuvered his way in and out of groups of students, house officers, nurses, and visitors like a miniature speed-demon. I could almost see him seated in a super racing car weaving through traffic and screeching its tires. He seemed utterly unaware of the paraphernalia attached to his small body, the tubes and bags flapping wildly, and threatened to fall or collide at any moment while careening around chirping and laughing. He became for me a kind of icon, a place mark, though I didn't even know who he was, what was wrong with him, why he was there, or how long he would be hospitalized. But he seemed very much at home and seemed to know the precise moment when rounds began. For just as the several small patient-care teams, with me in one or another of them, would start out from the nurse's station on daily rounds, there he'd be, getting in everyone's way and having a ball doing it. He was clearly loved by everyone, and no one ever complained.

One of the pediatricians who made rounds with us, Mark, lean and angular with a gait you could detect a mile away ("Hey, there's Mark, couldn't be anybody else, not with the way those knees and elbows are flapping!"), asked me one day if I would like to attend a patient-care conference; I readily agreed. It was scheduled for the next day, and he mentioned in passing that a lot of people would be there and that I might find the conference quite interesting.

Just before 10:00 the next morning, when the meeting was supposed to begin, I went up to the conference room and peeked in. It seemed that the room was already full with at least fifteen people seated; I thought I had come in on another meeting that was just concluding. But as I slowly backed out thinking I was in the wrong place, I noticed Mark seated at the other end gesturing for me to come on in. I went in, a bit puzzled at the crowd since it was still not quite 10:00; I had already learned that conferences do not start early in hospitals. I soon found out the pressing nature of this gathering.

As soon as I sat down, a physician at the head of the table began talking, as if my entrance were the signal for "go." Apparently they were waiting for me. I listened and began taking notes. The case sounded awfully familiar; it was the "hallway kid" they were talking about. Things didn't sound at all good. Even though much of the technical lingo was still beyond me, it was plain that things were not going well, and everyone there had the kind of bleak expression that confirmed it. As I listened it gradually dawned on me that this lovely child was going to die very soon, and nothing could be done about it.

With a shard of ice up my spine, I listened and gradually began to piece together the awful picture. Born at another hospital, this boy had massive problems from the outset, something called "short-gut" syndrome. He was born with only a tiny segment of functional intestine; the rest was dead, necrotic. Faced with this, the first response had been surgery to take out the bad and leave in the good, hoping that in time it would gradually stretch and function enough to allow growth. In his case, the remaining good gut was so small (as I recall, it was only about 7 centimeters) that it simply could not expand enough to function for the entire gut. He thus had to have a central line placed, with a catheter for feeding. In every other respect, this beautiful boy was perfectly normal.

About two and a half at the time of the conference, he had been continuously hospitalized since birth. The periodic attempts at weaning him from the central line to see if oral feeding could be managed had all failed: the tiny piece of gut just couldn't stretch enough to allow him to take in nourishment by mouth. When it became clear that this wasn't working, when he would get close to death by starvation, they would have to reinstitute the tube feeding. He would spring back, and in a short time was as active as ever; then, more time on tube feeds, then back to the trial at oral feeding, and back again. I wondered how long this sort of thing could go on.

I had no more than thought that question than the answer came from the physician reviewing his case. "Finite." You could keep this up for only a finite amount of time before the veins into which the nourishment was being fed by tube would collapse and couldn't be used again. So, another vein had to be found, but it, too, would eventually collapse. And, it turned out, they were at the end of their rope, for the "finite amount of time" had suddenly become starkly real. This marvelous little kid was going to die soon despite every effort—routine, investigational, and experimental. Nothing could be done to stop the inevitable.

The physician abruptly stopped talking. Silence. If a leaf had fallen, it could have been heard. My growling stomach sounded so loud I was sure that that was what brought all those eyes to me, for as I looked up from my notes and doodles I was greeted with faces turned toward me, eyes looking at me with expectation.

"Dr. Zaner, what do you think we should do?"

At the meeting were the attending physician, the surgeon who had done the initial surgery, several residents and interns, the primary-care nurses from several shifts, the head nurse, the unit's social worker, a child psychiatrist, several interested pediatricians (including Mark), the unit's dietitian, and me. Everyone, it seemed, knew the case, and many of them knew the little boy very well, having served in one or another way over the course of the past several years. Only I was new to situation. And, they wanted me to talk, to say something. I was, it became painfully clear, the agenda for the conference.

At the time, all I could think of was how much I didn't know, so naturally that's what prompted my first reaction: "Who, and where, are the parents?" I asked. "Surely they have a substantial stake here." Immediately, several of the nurses began to talk about the parents. It seemed that this was one of the problems. The parents, we were told, had for some time become increasingly absent; their visits were fewer and the time they spent when they did come was briefer. When they were there, they had less and less to say to anyone. They would go into Johnny's room and sit, staring blankly, saying very little while he kept up his active, running patter. Increasingly, the nurses noted that it was difficult to reach them or get them to talk. Then the attending spoke up, remarking that he hadn't really seen the parents in over three months; but the last time he had seen them, they were already becoming reticent and unresponsive to questions. This was confirmed by several residents who, during their respective rotations, had noted the same thing. The social worker also spoke, again confirming the apparent retreat from involvement. Then, the surgeon remarked that he had not yet even met the parents. Puzzled by all this, I thought it important to pursue the matter further. But first, something else had been nagging at the corners of my mind, and I decided to plunge ahead.

Something about the way the boy's condition had been presented bothered me, and I needed to be clear about it. "Johnny is dying, right?" Yes. "And nothing can be done to prevent it?" Yes. "How will he die? From not eating? From starvation?" Yes—which will be excruciating for everyone, especially for Johnny and his parents. "So," I blundered ahead, "it seems to me that what you're really saying is that you'd like, if at all possible, to find a way to ease that death, to shorten his pain and suffering." And, even more blunderingly, "Isn't what you really want to know is whether it's possible to help him die? Now, if that's the point, then aren't you suggesting some form of active euthanasia?"

At the mere mention of that awful, awesome word, the straining tension broke, its fragile spring wound too tight. Suddenly, everyone started talking, spouting, rather, denying that anything like that could possibly be on anyone's mind. Emphatic, decisive, hard, and harsh denial. No, that awful thing was criminal and beyond the pale. But, the breaking of the tight tension also brought out other things, things that I thought were very significant.

While Johnny was going to die, inevitably and inexorably from his inability to take in nutrition because tube feeding had become impossible to continue, much could and would be done to ease that process through the control of pain and other palliative measures. And while the process would take time, this gradual sinking into death would be accompanied by natural body processes which themselves would, thankfully, probably help and even ease the process, making it less gruesome than otherwise. But most significantly, I had really asked the wrong question. Though this wasn't stated in so many words, it became very clear that the real issue was not how he would die, not even what would be the cause of death nor how long it would take. The issue that riveted and stabbed at them was where he would die.

Everything zeroed in on that "where?" from then on. As the parents had become gradually less and less involved, quite naturally those who were with Johnny most often and most intimately, especially the primary-care nurses, had effectively bonded with him, to the point that they seemed even to resent the parents and took the parents' apparent lack of concern quite personally. Even the attending seemed bound up with the child in a more personal way than I had witnessed before. "Taking care of" Johnny had shifted into "caring for" Johnny.

With the tension loosened, a complete picture began to emerge. It appeared that these parents, both still in their twenties and Johnny their first child, were not only somewhat naive and immature, but at the same time truly shattered by everything that had been going on since Johnny was born. After all, they had never had him at home, they had had to arrange visits around their other activities, and they seemed to understand that there was no hope for their child. They were already grieving, already going through a profound loss experience. They had, in effect, been going through this for several years and thus were suffering prolonged and protracted grief and loss.

Further probing revealed an even more complex story, one that did not come out until after the attending physician and surgeon had met with the young couple. Each of the parents came from families who were deeply involved in what were described as "fundamentalist" religious sects, though not the same ones. The husband's father was a preacher in one, and the mother's mother a preacher in the other. To add to the complications, both of the young parents had been seen as prodigals to their respective families; when it became known that the pregnancy had occurred before marriage, they were subjected to serious criticisms from both sides. Even more, when the baby was born and its problems known, the parents were informed that this was "God's punishment" for their sins. Little wonder, we all thought when this story became known, that these young people had been acting oddly. They had to contend with their child's condition and continuous hospitalization, their own sense of having possibly done something to make it happen, and then the constant accusations from both families that they had indeed been sinful and made to suffer God's wrath.

Although I was not able to meet the parents, reports from those who did were very revealing. It seems that when they were encouraged to talk about themselves, the flood of conflicting feelings came rushing out. And, no sooner did that happen than they began to feel far more capable of grappling with the truth of their child's dismal future. They made it clear that they desperately wanted to have Johnny home during his final days. This was arranged, without complaint from any of the care team, which now also had come to a fuller appreciation and understanding. They took him home where he managed to survive for a few months, even managing to take in some oral feeding, though it was insufficient to sustain life. He then died peacefully in their arms. A letter from the couple expressed their deep gratitude for having been enabled to express themselves and have the time with their son.

Some time later Mark stopped me in the hallway and expressed his and the care team's "profound thanks" for what I did. At the time, I was puzzled. "What in the world are you talking about?" I asked. "What 'help' do you mean?"

"Don't you remember that conference about Johnny?" Mark returned.

"Johnny? What did I do there?" All I recalled doing was little more than repeating what I had heard those folks themselves say.

Mark's profuse gratitude caught me by complete surprise; I couldn't figure out what he could be talking about. He pointed out that the attending, the surgeon, and the others were themselves surprised by what I had said. They had suddenly realized that they had been taking it for granted that they faced one issue, the "where?" question. When they realized that the parents' apparent retreat might be resolvable, they then understood the crucial need to have a very candid discussion with them. As the result of that discussion, the heretofore caretakers were able to release him confidently to his parents, now known to be very caring.

Reflecting on the letter from Johnny's parents, the team realized that the impact of "ethical" decision making extended beyond the patient-provider relationship. What happened there, and has occurred in numerous conferences and encounters since, was not so much something I did as it was something I allowed to happen. Maybe it was even bound to occur. This was the first time these particular physicians and nurses and others had sat down to listen to an "ethicist," and it served more as a sort of forum for—even an endorsement of—a kind of conversation that was unusual for them. Regardless of how each of them variously understood "ethics," the sheer fact of including me in their conference served to legitimate topics that, for many of them, had not been thought appropriate before. "All I did was repeat what I heard them saying, after all," as I told Mark. "What I heard them saying" turns out to have been the critical thing.

As I think about things now, using the awful word "euthanasia" struck them to the quick; and while this may well have been on their minds, its open mention was enough to make the conversation shift ground immediately and drastically. It served to force a kind of basic reconsideration of what they had been saying and thus refocus what was really on their minds. On the other hand, close on the loud denials, the queries about these parents brought out how little they in fact knew about them, and the immediate need to find out more. In my subsequent work it has become clear that there are hitherto-taboo topics within the confidential confines of the physician-patient relationship that really do have to be discussed with increasing openness and candor. By addressing awesome and deeply troubling topics like physician-assisted suicide and euthanasia, it becomes possible to discover critical underlying concerns.

As I now reflect on what went on in that conference, it was exactly the mention of that forbidden topic of euthanasia that triggered a kind of resolving response. Under all that talk—and, yes, even denial—what was deeply feared was that Johnny would have to go through a really awful death. Buried beneath all the talk of the "where?" question was the urgent hope that he would at least have a good death, which is essentially what euthanasia is all about.

And yet while that seems to have been the underlying theme of those conversations, it could not be openly discussed. Indeed, not even afterwards, when that "good death" was in fact what actually occurred, could this topic be openly discussed. Now, of course, things have changed somewhat. There has been the publicity generated around Dr. Jack Kevorkian—"Dr. Death"—and his "Death Machine." There was also the more recent publication in a major medical journal of another case where a patient's physician helped her to die, "assisted suicide," as it's been termed, as well as another where the physician found he simply could not do that. There has even been somewhat more open discussion of euthanasia thanks to the efforts of various groups that support it and to the greater openness with which euthanasia has been accepted in the Netherlands.

And so, that more caring resolution, that good death that came to Johnny in the loving embrace of his parents, was not so much due to anything I directly contributed to the treatment team as it was my serving as a sort of catalyst. Now more widely known as "decision facilitator," this role opened up a whole new world for understanding the role of clinical ethics for them and for me. I began to realize that there are times when, even if the ethicist cannot offer direct advice or recommendations, being present as an ethicist is of itself a trigger for very crucial conversations.

This role is rarely addressed in the circles of philosophy in relation to medical and clinical ethics even though, truth be told, that is very much what teaching is about: helping others to think more carefully about their circumstances, the options and decisions they must face, the responsibility these decisions carry with them, and the need to consider, among available options, which are really most congruent or harmonious with each individual's basic sense of what is worthwhile—a key part of what morality is all about. There may be method to this madness, but it is surely quite different from what many think ethics is all about. All things considered, clinical ethics is turning out to be deeply satisfying and intriguing—hopefully, even therapeutic in its way.

# F I V E

# Accidents and Time:
# The Urge to Be Normal

Recently I received a call from a physician who wanted me to stop by
to see a young man who had been hospitalized and was refusing
hemodialysis. Refusal of treatment meant death. The patient was in
his late twenties, and he had been hospitalized numerous times the
previous summer for all manner of problems and was apparently just
fed up with everything.

Reading his chart, I was stunned. This young man's life seemed
to thread out from an infancy I had encountered many times before
with premature babies in the NICU. He had been born with spina
bifida, making him paraplegic and hydrocephalic, and had a surgi-
cally implanted shunt that took the cerebral-spinal fluid from his
brain to his abdomen and, like any of such children who survive and
manage to grow, had undergone repeated surgeries over the years to
replace the shunt. He was also incontinent with permanent reliance
on a bag outside his body to collect the accumulated urinary fluid.

That summer he had began to suffer from severe diarrhea,
dehydration, infections, and a malfunctioning bladder and was
repeatedly hospitalized. As if all that were not enough, his kidneys
had begun to fail and he had become anemic. Now, hospitalized
again, he staunchly refused to have dialysis even though it held the

promise of at least some benefit, even a return to home and possibly the job he had held for some years. His physician, thinking that the young man was experiencing depression, prescribed an antidepressant hoping that he might, in a less distressed state, change his mind.

The patient had been brought to the hospital by his mother, who expected that he would be placed on hemodialysis; maybe even at some point, she thought, he might have a kidney transplant. But as soon as he was admitted he began refusing dialysis. Fortunately for those in charge, he didn't need immediate dialysis, so it was easy to postpone things and start the antidepressant. Then, when he changed his mind, as was fully expected, they could put a catheter into his arm through which he would then be periodically hooked to the machine and the toxins that his kidneys could no longer manage would be mechanically removed. But despite the antidepressant, he continued to refuse dialysis. Within a few days, the poisons inevitably built up and dialysis was seriously needed. His mother was terrified. His physician had gone out of town for the weekend and the resident and nurses seemed at loggerheads with this patient's persistent refusal.

In the press of circumstances, the physician covering for the attending decided to have a psychiatrist assess his competence. Surely, it was thought, no one in his right mind would refuse treatments that promised relief and return to normalcy. Unsurprisingly, by that time the psychiatrist found him "temporarily incompetent," and his "decision against dialysis" was taken to be a function of depression and failing thought processes, said to be caused by the build-up of poisons in his bloodstream. Armed with that, the covering physician was able to place the catheter and take him off to be dialyzed.

When the attending returned he was quite concerned—furious is probably more accurate. Not only had his patient been dialyzed despite refusing it the previous week, but here the young man was alert once again—the dialysis had, after all, done its thing—and very disturbed at being forced to have dialysis. In fact, he continued his adamant refusal of any further sessions with the dialysis machine.

Both the attending and his mother were in a bind: both wanted to respect what they considered to be the young man's competently expressed refusal though knowing that dialysis was actually beneficial. But he said that he had had enough, in fact a lifetime of enough.

After hearing the plight of this young man, I remembered a patient from earlier in my career. Dax Cowart, a burn victim, unsuccessfully refused treatment and became something of a *cause célèbre*. Intended solely for educational purposes, a video of his hospitalization and forced treatment became a rallying point for individuals and groups concerned with promoting the idea that people have a right to refuse medical treatments even when they are likely to be beneficial. The doctrine of informed consent had at that time only begun to be accepted when using human beings as research subjects, but it was not generally thought to have application for treatments that were known to be beneficial.

After college and service in the Air Force as a jet pilot, Don Cowart (he later changed his name to "Dax") had joined his father's real estate business. One day they parked their car in a depression by a creek while they checked out a piece of property. When they got ready to leave, however, the car would not start. Don stayed in the driver's seat while his father checked out the engine. When he tried to start it, sparks from the engine set off a massive explosion. Fire engulfed the surrounding landscape. His father was thrown some distance away, and Don was trapped behind the steering wheel. He received third-degree burns over 65 percent of his body. His father was barely alive when Don struggled out of the car to get to him. Amazingly, though his eyes were badly burned and severe pain seared through his already charred body, Don was able to run through three walls of fire and up a dirt road about a half mile before he collapsed at the roadside. Hearing a man's footsteps, he was able to send the farmer back to find his father. When the man returned, Don asked him to bring a gun so that he could finish what the explosion and fire had almost done to him. The man refused, having already called for an ambulance, and Don was taken with his father to an intensive care unit of a major referral center 140 miles away. Don's father did not survive.

Then, as at the roadside, Don wanted to be left alone to die. Indeed, he adamantly demanded to be allowed to die. At the medical center he begged his physicians to let him die. He pleaded with his mother and lawyer to be discharged from one hospital after another so that he could kill himself, all the time raging against the excruciatingly painful treatments and the "insensitive" doctors, nurses, and orderlies. None would consent to his demands, and he remained hospitalized for the next fourteen months, receiving treatments until he was able to be discharged to his mother's care. Languishing for several years after, Dax still insists that he was right in his demands and that he was wronged in being forced to undergo treatment against his refusal, even though he has managed to reconstruct much of his life and even to find new love and be married.

When I agreed to the dialysis consult, thoughts of Dax were spinning through my mind. And not only Dax, but all those babies I had come to know in the NICU. It was as if one of them had grown up and was now demanding to know why he had been forced to stay alive. Until now I had only been able to wonder what the future held for those many babies. Well, here it was, Mr. Thomas Pembroke Brown, my very own anticipated worst fear come to life. Except, like most worst fears come to life, he proved to be very little like what I had imagined. Reality makes fools of us all.

When I went into his room, his mother was sitting next to his bed. Thomas was lying with his eyes closed, as if asleep. I said hello to his mother and introduced myself, but before I could say anything else, Thomas opened his eyes, said hello, and the barriers that had unwittingly been constructed in my mind collapsed. He looked and sounded *normal*. Discussion with the attending and notes in Tom's chart led me to focus on issues about death. It seemed to me that Tom and his mother needed to think and talk about death, too. I wondered whether they had in fact done much thinking about what would inevitably happen should he not have dialysis. Did he know, as his mother surely did, that refusing treatment would bring about *his* death?

After some small talk with them, I turned to Tom to try to open that sensitive topic. Suddenly his eyes rolled up and he began gagging and twitching and his face contorted. I quickly called in his nurse, who calmly took charge, informing me that Tom was going through a seizure. Clearly not a time to start a conversation about death and dying, I took my leave. I expressed my concern and apologies to his mother and promised to come back the next day.

I was really shaken as I walked away from his room. This was the first time I had witnessed a grand mal seizure in person and I was deeply troubled. My thoughts and feelings were turbulent. I even found myself foolishly wondering whether I had brought it on. As I later found out when I talked to his doctor, everyone had become so centered on Tom's refusal of dialysis that they had forgotten to tell me that, after years of being effectively controlled, his seizures had recently returned. As if everything else that he had endured over the past few months was not enough, now he had to contend with that. Thinking about that, I must say that his refusal of dialysis began to take on greater weight. But realizing that natural tendencies can be naturally misleading, I worked to mute that inclination.

The next morning I came back to see Tom and his mother. Things were much calmer and we moved directly to the issues at hand. Did he understand the implications of his refusal of dialysis? In a way, he did; but as we talked it seemed to me that he hadn't thought it out at all well. He was in fact behaving rather differently than one would expect when meeting someone firmly refusing potentially life-saving treatment. It's not that he was calmly accepting. He had not in fact discussed the matter with his mother; he had not really even thought about it much for himself. He had not signed any advanced directive; the idea hadn't even occurred to him. And his mother had not raised the issue with him of the advanced directive or the clear consequence of his refusal. The thought that he would die without dialysis had, so to speak, sort of sidled past his awareness now and then, but he had not confronted matters squarely. And his mother had not made her own feelings explicit to him.

Trying to learn more about Tom personally, I asked him about his job, one which he obviously enjoyed and in which he took some pride. It was an office-type position with a state agency, and it had given him a good deal of independence. Before he became so sick some months ago, he had even started to think he could get his own apartment and begin to live on his own. *That*, it seemed to me, was what was really on his mind. The numerous illnesses and hospitalizations had eventually required him to quit his job, which more than anything else seemed the source of his depression. Like all of us at one time or another, he had it all "figured out": on dialysis he would not be able to hold a job, much less go back to the one he really liked— *ergo*, life ain't worth it, so let's just give up. Being "normal," working and living independently, had become an insurmountable goal when viewed from his perspective.

He continued talking and I listened. A few months ago, he said, almost as an afterthought, he had been told by his supervisor that his job would be waiting for him when he was able to return. As soon as he said this he noticeably perked up; his talk became more lively, his gestures more animated.

"That's right," his mother quickly affirmed, "Mrs. Y did say you could have your job back when you're able."

"But how can I work," Tom's tremulous words seemed at once hopeful and wary, "when I've got to be on that damned machine so much?"

His mother and I vied with each other to get the thing said: work was indeed possible. Hadn't he discussed this with his doctor? He wasn't sure. Perhaps he had been so wrapped up in grief and a deep sense of loss that he hadn't heard. Or perhaps none of his doctors had thought to mention it or, if any of them had, Tom hadn't understood. In any event, it was clear that the way things appeared had changed dramatically for him. I suggested that he really needed to find out much more about dialysis and to call up his supervisor to check with her about returning to work. The conversation then wound down. It was perfectly obvious that he did not want to refuse dialysis and that he desperately wanted to get out of the hospital and back to work. It was then necessary to set up meetings with his doctor, who would be able to help him arrange a convenient place for outpatient treatment and, eventually, help him be evaluated for a transplant.

Before things concluded, I felt the need to bring some resolution to the issue that had brought me into his life in the first place: his refusal of treatment. I wanted to emphasize how important it was for him to confront that issue. Both he and his mother needed candid and continuous talk about death—especially the need for him to set out his wishes clearly. After all, he was still not well. He remained seriously ill. He might in fact find himself once again in the hospital and, perhaps, unable at that time to voice his wishes. It would be unfortunate were that to happen and for his mother to find herself in a situation in which she did not know what he would want done, or not done.

We talked about the matter for a bit, including some discussion of the new state law on advance directives, do-not-resuscitate orders, withholding and withdrawing of life-supports—the whole gamut of issues his medical condition might well bring about. I mentioned, too, how deeply affected I had been by those tiny babies in the NICU, especially what happened to them after they were discharged, and shared my apprehensions about first meeting him. Then I left, thanking him and his mother for allowing me into their lives under such difficult circumstances and emphasizing how much they had helped me understand.

As I was walking out, Tom called out, "Hey, doc, what do you *really* do for a living? How do you make your bucks?"

"I guess you could say that I'm a teacher, a college prof, Tom. Only, my students are medical students, young doctors, attending physicians, nurses—even patients and families, people like you and your mother." This situation was a first for me. It's still the only one I've encountered since Dax in which a patient has refused treatments that are beneficial. (Many patients who are terminally ill refuse treatments that are futile.) I found it deeply disturbing, even though

I had discussed Dax Cowart's situation with Dax and with others many times. Tom, like Dax, was surely competent to decide things for himself. He had in fact done so several times. That he was depressed is surely true, although it could be disputed whether it was psychiatric in nature, thus permitting that override of his wishes. That he needed to be confronted with the consequences of his decision was doubtless also true—or was my presumption only an expression of my own anxiety and denial?

The plain fact is that I remain uncertain, and questions continue to haunt me. When Tom first expressed his refusal to undergo dialysis, shouldn't that have had priority? Did his decline into renal psychosis change the competency with which he chose that condition? The decline, after all, was exactly what one would expect to occur. Within a day or so, he would have lapsed into an irreversible coma and then died. And wasn't this just what he had chosen? By the time I got involved he had already had one course of dialysis, had improved considerably, and was still adamantly expressing his refusal of treatment. Shouldn't his decision have prevailed? What business did I have going in there and talking about living wills, do-not-resuscitate orders, and death? Wasn't that, for all my attempts to be understanding and helpful, just another form of coercion? Thinking about that brings to mind something else. If it was proper to call the psychiatrist on the weekend, wasn't it also appropriate to have him visit Tom on Monday, when he again refused dialysis? And, if so, why ask for an ethics consult?

Or, consider an alternate possibility. Was a psychiatrist needed at *any* point? Living as we do under the umbrella of autonomy, the principal norm of our form of individualism, if Tom was "competent" to make his own decisions early in the week, then there seems no question but that it was his right to make whatever decisions he wished. Shouldn't that have closed the issue? Once a competent person chooses for him or herself, the game is over for the rest of us, whatever we ourselves may or may not do in similar circumstances and whether we like what Tom decided or not. By what right, then, could anyone else contradict Tom's choice?

Then there is his mother. He didn't seem concerned with what his decision was doing to his mother. Perhaps that should have been the theme of my discussion with him. Perhaps talking about death did provoke something in him. Maybe it caused him to think of things he hadn't considered before—his mother, job, relationships with other people, and the life he really wanted to have but couldn't see well enough through such dark lenses and so many recent trips to the hospital.

The last time I visited Tom he was on the dialysis machine. He told me that his boss had told him that he could have his old job back. He was very upbeat, joshing about the machine, joking with his nurse, and offering to come to one of my classes and talk about himself. I didn't have the heart then—maybe I didn't have the courage—to ask him why he had earlier refused to be precisely where he now was. Nor do I have whatever it would take to ask him now. Maybe later, when he (or I) has had time to think about things, when time can work its subtle alchemistry on our memories and deepest feelings about ourselves . . . then, perhaps, I can ask. In the meantime,

*I suppose there might have been a time*
*—a time of apples and children*
   *of women and glances*
   *of rain, snow and wild winds—*
*When things now usual and plain*
*Were only themselves, shining;*
*When in innocence we could let them be,*
*As be they might, driven in on our eyes*
*Like eagles, or in silence shared awhile*
*With no need of words . . .*
*Beneath a sheath of trees. . . .*
*A time of talking and whispering together*
*Like faintly shifting leaves.*
*Or singing slipping through the quiet air*
*Like birds' wings,*
*With minds like picnics spread quietly around*
*A mound of soft grass.*
*If such times of knowing (being) are*

*What it's all about, then what is time?*
*Quick paradox of inwardness: yearning*
*On the further edge of living, for what was,*
*And ought to be, or have been. . . .*
*To whom offer these sly celebrations of memory?*
*On whom depend for understanding where we stand,*
*Beneath the bows of trees, lying, on our backs,*
*Thinking of home and apples, children and glances,*
*Listening for voices, like birds sleeping in leaves,*
*To tell us, now, in this needful time, the time we are,*
*Who we are, or why?*

I'm not sure why Tom remains so firmly in my mind. Neither deft nor subtle, he was in truth, and I'm sure remains, unvarnished. It is not so much his refusal that stands out as the harsh accident of his birth. That utterly fortuitous and subtle genetic accident that destined this gentle, artless individual to face, unasked, a life strident with curious and unaccountable nostalgia. Yearning to be *normal*.

S   I   X

# Life Can Never Be the Same

One of the units I work with quite a bit is maternal-fetal medicine in the Department of Obstetrics and Gynecology. Like a few other units around the country, ours offers practically every kind of prenatal diagnosis: ultrasonography, amniocentesis, fetoscopy, chorionic villus sampling (CVS)[1]—the works. Problems of all sorts can be detected very early in pregnancy.

This subspecialty of obstetrics has been changing rapidly and can be expected to continue rapid advancement from discoveries coming out of the Human Genome Project. One of the most ambitious and important scientific ventures of this century, this project seeks to map all of the human body's genes numbering between 50,000 and 100,000 and containing the blueprints for the thousands of proteins that make up the body's tissues and vital organs. One of its direct consequences, as I've learned on more than one occasion, is the possibility of genetic testing to determine whether a developing baby is afflicted with one of the thousands of genetic diseases that affect people. While treatment still lies very much in the future, *diagnosis* is already at hand for many of these problems. The aim of prenatal diagnosis is to detect genetic and congenital diseases as well as structural problems. The hope is that diagnosis can improve the chances of having a healthy baby at birth by providing important information for making decisions during pregnancy.

Perhaps most significant to the development of maternal-fetal medicine is diagnostic ultrasonography, the dominant technique both for visualizing the fetus in utero and for enhancing the safety and effectiveness of other, more invasive, diagnostic techniques like amniocentesis or fetoscopy. Not too long ago, another diagnostic tool was developed that broadens therapeutic options and allows for safer and more accurate and rapid determination of fetal well being, Percutaneous Umbilical Blood Sampling (PUBS). This technique involves obtaining samples of fetal blood. Guided by ultrasonography, a needle is positioned and inserted to draw blood from the fetus's umbilical artery where it goes into the placenta. After blood is drawn and tested to make sure it is fetal blood, it can be analyzed in as little as forty-eight hours. Results of the test can harbor important information for many different actual and potential problems such as blood disorders, neurological problems, and many others that occur due to genetic or congenital flaws in development. Within two days one can be presented with some really difficult problems—which I was to learn when I was asked to see a couple who had been referred to the maternal-fetal unit for evaluation.

"You know," Mrs. Albert told me, "I really didn't have any idea why you came in to see me that first time. Not that you weren't nice and all, but, really, I couldn't figure it. But later on, that next time, and then when you met with Bob and me about the test results, it was sure good to be able to talk with someone we knew. I mean, after that first time failed—I was more awake and heard more, I think, than the doctors thought, you know?—and then, well, they wanted to do it again . . . well, that was really hard, heavy you know? Bob and me, well, we didn't know what we should do, and it was good having someone there—you, I mean—to talk about it. It really helped to get things straighter. But then, after that second test failed, too, things really fell apart for us; I mean, who would have thought that the damned thing, that catheter, would just slip out again, the same way it had the first time? Of course, putting the needle in did help the baby, it did drain the bladder again, but then . . ." Her voice trailed off, submerged in still-vivid memories, suffused with emotions of that time more than a year before when I had last seen her.

She had been referred by her physician to the maternal-fetal unit for evaluation of a problem that he thought he had detected on ultrasound in his office several days before. As best as could be estimated, she was about fourteen or fifteen weeks into her pregnancy. The couple had not planned to get pregnant but had welcomed the news when it came. She had had excellent prenatal care, part of which included an ultrasound. Her obstetrician wanted to see how things were going and, among other things, to determine the fetus's gestational age. What he saw was not comforting. He couldn't be sure what it was, but of this he was certain: something was not right. He strongly urged her to come to our unit for evaluation.

Just before she scheduled the visit, I had begun seeing a special group of obstetric patients. PUBS had just been started and, realizing its potential, I wanted to see whether early and continuous discussions with an ethicist would be at all helpful for patients as well as for physicians and nurses. Although PUBS had been in use for some time in England and France, one of our obstetricians had only recently been to England to learn how to do it and was anxious to determine its effectiveness here.

When I met Mrs. Albert, I had already seen several other patients scheduled for the test. I felt that I was only beginning to get a feel for the potent issues it implied. Mrs. Albert's visit, however, quickly put things in perspective. Her physician had referred her because he thought he had seen a large cystic mass in the fetus's abdomen. This was confirmed by our ultrasonographer. It was thought that the fetus's kidneys were okay, but a severe blockage in the bladder was preventing expulsion of urine into the amniotic fluid. This posed several problems. The already seriously distended bladder could not expand much further without damage to the bladder wall and the surrounding internal organs. Moreover, the resulting decreased amniotic fluid would eventually cause damage to the fetal lungs (pulmonary dysplasia), as lung development depends on sufficient amniotic fluid. Without intervention it was probable that the fetus would not survive beyond a few weeks. In one-fourth of known cases with similar problems, other anomalies have been found and the prognosis for these fetuses is dismal. Being informed of this, Mrs. Albert was encouraged to agree to other tests. These included karyotyping to see whether the problems were genetic in origin.

I told Mrs. Albert and her husband that a team of people would be meeting shortly to figure out what, if anything, was going on and what might be done. Neither said very much at that time; they were very anxious. "We'll just have to wait to see what they find out," Mr. Albert said. Since the attending physician had already discussed the problems with them, they knew full well that things didn't look at all good. They pointed out to me, though, that they did not believe in abortion and hoped that something could be worked out.

A team conference was held to review findings, and several options were discussed. As the fetus was only fourteen-weeks gestational age at the time, the pregnancy could be terminated; but that phrase, I thought, was not altogether accurate. "What we're talking about," I emphasized, "is abortion—therapeutic abortion, to be sure, but from what Mr. and Mrs. Albert told me, they might be opposed to that." Still, the team insisted that, however worded, this was an option that needed to be presented and discussed with them. A PUBS procedure could be done to determine whether there was an abnormal karyotype, which might also indicate if other anomalies were present, though they could not yet be visualized on ultrasound. If there was a genetic problem, the couple would have additional information and might then opt either to continue with the pregnancy or to abort and try for another pregnancy. After the PUBS, which was felt to be necessary in any case, a fetal surgical procedure could be done to implant a tiny Harrison Shunt into the fetal bladder to drain it into the amniotic cavity. If successful, it would then be recommended that Mrs. Albert be kept in the hospital for some time for continuous care and evaluation.

It was eventually agreed that the PUBS procedure recommendation was most reasonable and would be offered. Any subsequent decision could then be made based on what was found. If the karyotype turned out normal, the fetal surgery would then be offered. If the karyotype was abnormal, indicating a serious genetic anomaly, a therapeutic abortion would be offered on the basis that the risks to her and to her pregnancy seemed to outweigh the benefits of the shunt procedure for the baby. Depending on what the couple decided, other decisions would be faced.

The PUBS was offered, and the couple agreed. They felt that it would give them the kind of information they would need in order to know what to do. Before the PUBS was done the next day, a genetic counselor met with them. Later that evening, I went back to see them again, as I wanted to make sure that they really understood not only what the PUBS might show but also what options they might then face. Mr. Albert was not there when I went into Mrs. Albert's room. She was very clear about what she had been told. She was also very worried about the risks of the procedure for her baby. She knew that PUBS was new, less tried, and that while many of the risks to her and to her baby of a surgical procedure were known, its long-term effects were still somewhat uncertain. She was right to be worried. Even though in England and France it had been found to be statistically no more risky than amniocentesis, this seemed mainly a matter of the surgeon's experience, and it had not been done many times in the United States. Though others were scheduled, this would be one of the first times PUBS had been done at this center. Still, the skill for the technique is pretty much the same as what is needed for amniocentesis, and the physician doing PUBS had done that many times.

"I know," she told me. "I just want to talk about it; it helps to hear yourself thinking out loud, if you know what I mean. . . . I mean, from what the doctor told me, he's going to try to put a small, hollow needle into my baby's umbilical artery, where it goes into the placenta, right?"

"That's what I understand," I said.

"But that's just a tiny, tiny, little thing! How's he going to get a needle into that? I mean, I have a hard time getting thread through my sewing needle! I know what they're trying to do, but it just seems so strange." After we talked it over some more, she told me that she had already decided to "go for it," as it seemed that she didn't have many other choices.

"You know, though," I reminded her, "that you could decide for abortion."

"I know, but that doesn't seem right, not if there is a chance something can be done."

"Don't forget, Mrs. Albert, all these choices and decisions are yours—yours and your husband's—and nobody else's. You could decide not to have PUBS done at any time, even when you're lying there on the operating table. You know, just the other day that happened. A lady was scheduled for PUBS and, at the very last minute—she had already been prepped and was partially anesthetized, and she just sat right up and said 'No, I don't want this done.'"

"Really? What happened?"

"They stopped. It was her decision, and this is your decision. You can decline at any moment and nobody's going to do anything you don't want, and nobody's going to think the worse of you if you back out. It's really important that you realize this."

As I was about to leave her room, she told me that she was still going through with it and that she would appreciate it if I would stop back when the results came in, only about forty-eight hours later. She was right to be worried about how tiny the umbilical artery was. This would be the first time in any center, here or abroad, that the procedure had been attempted on a fetus less than eighteen-weeks gestational age.

Before the PUBS was done, the fetus's bladder had to be drained to relieve the pressure. This was done by needle puncture using ultrasound for guidance. As was expected, the ultrasound taken draining the bladder showed that fluid was immediately reaccumulating, confirming the need to implant the shunt. In fact, two days later another ultrasound revealed that the bladder was distended and a small fissure had been caused by the needle puncture and had leaked fluid into the peritoneal cavity. If left alone, this could be a serious problem for other organs.

The results from the PUBS returned and everything was normal: no genetic anomalies. Only the obstructed bladder. The team met to discuss matters. Now, though, another controversy irrupted. One of the obstetricians expressed strong reservations about our offering "something so experimental" by physicians who were inexperienced with the procedure. Instead, he felt, the couple should be referred to a center where physicians had more experience. He also pointed out that implanting this shunt had never been done for a fetus this early in pregnancy, not even in England or France. The attending did not take the implied criticism well. A heated debate ensued, but the consensus of the group was that the procedure should at least be offered. Full information would also be offered that highlighted the very things that concerned this physician. The couple would also be told the risks and potential benefits of the procedure and, of course, other options, including the possibility of going to another center to have it done. It was noted, though, that if the couple elected to remain here the only other options were termination, which they opposed, or the status quo—"let nature take her course"—which meant that the fetus would eventually die in utero.

After the lively discussion, the consensus was to go ahead and offer what we could and let them decide. I was asked to talk it over with them again, as it was thought that someone slightly removed from the situation could best ensure more reasonable and defensible decisions. During my discussion with them it seemed to me that they fully understood the problems and prospects, the risks, benefits, and options. They again expressed strong opposition to abortion, but they did not want to undertake the two-thousand-mile trip to the other center, nor did they want to have to go through a procedure that would be done by complete strangers. They felt quite comfortable with their physicians and prospects here, and they wanted to have the "catheter thing" done here and done soon, as they knew that their baby's life was increasingly threatened with each passing day. Surgery was recommended by the attending, and they accepted the idea.

Mr. Albert and I were invited to observe the procedure and went together into the labor-and-delivery room. Mrs. Albert was already prepped; the ultrasonographer was almost ready to begin. Moving to a place where I could observe everything, I watched as what seemed a huge bladder came into view. The needle with the sheathed shunt was introduced through her stomach into her uterus and then through the fetal wall into the bladder. What incredible skill it took to place it just right and to get that tiny catheter with its butterfly valves at both ends, one going inside the bladder and the other outside, in the amniotic cavity just so. But as he began to withdraw the needle, something was clearly wrong: instead of staying in place, the catheter began to come out with the needle. Unable to get it back inside, there was no choice but to remove the entire thing.

The attending got on the phone right away to call the physician who had developed the shunt. I did not get to hear what was said, but several things were clear when he told me about the conversation. The shunt should have worked fine; the procedure using this shunt had been done over forty times already, and this was the first time this kind of glitch had been reported. He nevertheless agreed to supply another shunt, without charge. The attending was clearly disturbed and unsure just what to do now.

Mrs. Albert told me later that day that she had been partially alert during the process and had heard and understood what had happened. "Now what?" she wondered. "Is my baby going to die?"

I could only tell her that I just didn't know, but that she and Mr. Albert needed to talk it over with the attending. I mentioned that another team meeting would be held shortly to see what people think. "We did buy some time," I pointed out, "because even though the shunt came back out, it did succeed in draining the bladder again, and the doctor told me that there did not appear to be any further leakage from the puncture."

"I know," she said, "I heard him say that in the room." An amazing young woman, she even mentioned that she understood that "these things happen" sometimes and that "you just can't change it or do anything about it."

*Really amazing*, I thought to myself, for I had not witnessed a clearer expression of the fact that medicine is in the nature of the case subject to mistakes, not all of which are due to negligence. Some errors are not due to incompetence, nor to the state of the art; they simply happen. Nobody could have predicted that the shunt would not come off the needle like it was supposed to; it just happened.

The Alberts were, of course, disturbed—and not simply at the shunt's failure to stay in place. Now, after all, the same problem was still there: the fetus's bladder was still blocked and had refilled almost immediately after the puncture had drained it. "What do we do now?" Mr. Albert wanted to know. "The doctor mentioned that they could try it again. He said that the guy who invented that shunt told him that he was sending out another one right away. Should we do it again, like the doctor suggested? What if it fails again?"

I was a bit taken aback by this as the idea of a second attempt had not yet been discussed with me, yet here I was being asked without my knowing what had already been said to them. I had, in fact, thought that a second attempt was reasonable and should be offered, so I wasn't too disturbed by that news. This seemed to be a good time to encourage more discussion. I wondered what his wife thought about it, how she felt about things now, especially as she still faced the same situation. Her response was unequivocal: "Of course I'll try again! The doctor did everything right; it was just that damned shunt that didn't work right! We've *got* to give our baby the chance it deserves and I've already told the doctor that he has to try again. That doctor out in San Francisco said this type of thing had never happened before, didn't he? It's just a fluke."

Concerned that the first needle puncture not be a problem, the attending believed that at least a week was needed before the second effort could be made. She was checked again by ultrasound during that time and things seemed to be okay. Then, a week after the first attempt, she was again taken to labor-and-delivery and prepped. The second shunt had been carefully checked to make sure it was functioning correctly. The scene was repeated. The extended bladder came into view; the needle with its attached shunt was positioned and inserted; the attending's hands confidently moved the needle through her stomach, uterus, and into the fetal bladder, again draining the accumulated fluid. Positioned perfectly, he then slowly began the maneuver that was to release the shunt. You could see the butterfly tip extend inside the bladder. Then, as the needle was gradually retracted, the shunt could be seen to pull back. He tried to push it gently back into the bladder; it went back in. He again tried to withdraw the needle; back came the shunt. Something was wrong, for it was just not going to work. The shunt that had functioned outside the womb, for some reason would not function inside. Clearly dismayed and disgusted, the attending announced what was obvious to everyone there. "I don't care *what* San Francisco thinks or how many times it has worked with other patients, this design is just faulty. I'm withdrawing."

As happened the first time, Mrs. Albert was alert enough during this trial to know what was said. She, too, knew on fully awakening that the same thing had occurred. When I went in to see her a bit later, she was despondent. Her husband was angry.

"Now what?" he asked.

Addressing her husband, she said, "Now's no time to get mad. We've got to figure out what we do now, and anger won't help, you know?"

"Sure, I know," he responded, "but, dammit . . ."

"Don't curse, Tommie, please, not *now*." And, turning to me, "What do you think? What should we do now?"

What indeed, I wondered to myself. Before I could say anything, though, she said that the doctor had mentioned in passing several days before that if they wished they could still go to San Francisco and have the doctor there do open-uterine surgery.

What in the world's going on here? I ventured that they could do that if they wanted. "But do you understand what that involves?" I asked.

"Wait a minute, Sue," her husband burst out, "talk about something that's not been tried much. The nurse told me about that, that it's *really* experimental."

"I know, Tommie, but isn't it worth it?" And, again turning to me, "Isn't it, Dr. Zaner? I mean, what we've already been through is 'experimental,' isn't it?" She began weeping quietly.

Clearly this was no time to get into such a discussion, so I decided to let things rest a bit. "Why don't you let it sit a while; give it some time? I'll ask the doctor to talk to you about it. I will find out as much as I can about that surgery. For that matter, would you like *me* to get you more information about it? I'll find out what's available and see that you get it if you want. I don't think, though, that you should do anything until you've found out as much about that procedure as you did about PUBS and the shunt before you agreed to have them done. Just don't get into that business until you know more about it."

It seemed to me that they needed to be alone then, so I left. I went straight to the attending to find out for myself what he had said. He had mentioned the procedure, but only as a way of ensuring that all options had been at least discussed. He was not himself inclined, however, to recommend the open-uterine surgery. He said that it was just too experimental. They had only managed to do three or four of them—hardly enough to know the risks and benefits—unlike intra-uterine shunting, which had been tried at least forty or more times, and generally with good results.

"You need to let them know as much as you can about that," I pointed out, "since they are already thinking about it. Also, it might help to give them any pertinent literature you might have about the procedure. They got a great deal from what you shared with them about PUBS and the shunting procedure."

"Well," he answered, "there's really very little, if anything, in the literature about open-uterine surgical procedures to correct fetal defects. I'll certainly let them know everything I know about it and will give them my recommendation—that I would *not* recommend it at this time."

He was not particularly aware, I thought, of the irony in his remark: he had, after all, gone ahead with the PUBS with only little experience himself, and very little "in the literature." Now, he was not inclined to recommend the trip to San Francisco in large part because "the literature" didn't yet have many studies of the risks and benefits associated with open-uterine surgery. Interesting. He eventually agreed that it was only right to find out as much as he could about the risks and benefits of this surgery from the surgeon himself and to convey these candidly to the Alberts. If they really wished to know the attending's opinion, he was prepared to give it: he wouldn't recommend open-uterine surgery.

A meeting of the team was arranged the next day to review everything and decide what options could be presented to the couple. As the attending and I expected, nobody was willing to urge the couple to travel to San Francisco. But what could be recommended? As the discussion proceeded, therapeutic abortion increasingly loomed as the only option that could reasonably be offered. If nothing were done, after all, the baby's bladder would just keep on expanding, and displacing the other organs, and eventually the anomaly would kill it. What to do? Would it be the anomaly that killed it or us—the attending, the parents, and the rest of us being partners to the act? It was decided that therapeutic abortion had to be discussed with them, and I was requested to do it. The whole thing reduced to its core: this was their life, their decision, their choice.

Before I got back to them, the attending had responded candidly to all their questions about the possible risks and benefits of open-uterine surgery and had given them a couple of articles about it. When I went in, they were both there and greeted me with the question, one that was to haunt me ever since, and not only in connection with them. "When is enough enough?" Mrs. Albert asked. "I mean, you know, do we have to do that? Shouldn't we do it, for our baby?"

"How far does a person have to go?" Mr. Albert blurted out. "I mean, how do you know when you've done enough . . . done everything you can?"

"You know," I responded, "people, parents, inevitably wonder whether 'everything possible' has been done, whether there is ever any end to what 'might be done.' Like all of us, you only want to do the right thing, to do what is good for the baby. I know that. I also know that it's terribly hard to know what that "right" and "good" thing really is, especially in these circumstances. What can anybody say? What can *I* say? It's never easy to face that awful question. In a way, I suppose, you never know what you should include in that 'everything'—whether 'everything possible' includes just anything that even remotely could help. I don't know how remote something has to be for us to say you don't have to do it. . . ."

Mrs. Albert interrupted me. "But *is it worth it?* Can we live with ourselves if we *don't* do anything?"

"But, don't forget, Mrs. Albert, it's not as if you've done *nothing*. In fact, you've done a great deal already. Not once but *twice*, you've gone through attempts to correct your baby's problem; neither worked. That's not *nothing;* you have done a great deal. When you asked me if going to San Francisco would be *"worth it,"* all I can suggest is that you try and think about how far your responsibilities really extend. Does this include even agreeing to undergo a plainly experimental, even exotic, procedure where we just do not know what the benefits are, if any, and we *do* know a good deal about the risks? After all, we're talking about a serious piece of surgery known to carry considerable risks to you and doubtless the same for your baby. All things considered, I'd have to urge you to recognize that if you were to agree to go out there and have it done you would probably not be doing something that would in all likelihood help your baby, although it would doubtless be some benefit to other people. That surgeon, for instance, would learn much, especially about doing the procedure, which would add to scientific knowledge that could benefit other babies in the future. But is that something *you* should do? Do any of us have any obligation to contribute in that way—so to speak, to sacrifice ourselves for other people in this way?"

"When you put it that way," Mr. Albert said, "it looks quite different, and I'm not sure I understand."

"What I mean is that when you put everything together—the two attempts here to drain the urinary fluid, the unknowns about that other surgery, and the known risks of any surgical procedure to Mrs. Albert and to the baby—and you have to put everything together in *that* way, only then can you come to some reasonable moral conclusion about what it means to 'do everything possible.' I mean . . ."

"What you mean," Mrs. Albert broke in, "is that it's just not *worth* it, right? That we've already done enough? That 'going the extra mile' doesn't necessarily include something like straight-out experiments?"

What I meant, I went on to tell them, was that "doing everything" does have to be put into some sort of realistic context, that "reasonable options" do not have to include risky, experimental surgeries. Our moral responsibilities for our children, or children-to-be, are not unlimited, and I was urging them to think about this idea of *limits*. The way to get clearer about them is to try to weigh the most reasonable among the possible options. In this case, that was extremely difficult. This couple was deeply averse to the only other options: sit by and wait for the fetus to die *in utero* or undergo a therapeutic abortion. "The question you've got to decide is whether taking your chances with that surgery and risking both you and your baby is better than having an abortion and, after some time, trying to have another child."

"But that's *awful*," Mrs. Albert emphatically stated. "What do you do when *none* of the choices are good ones?"

I didn't know then, and I'm not sure I know now, just how to respond to that question. It is the kind of question that cuts to the moral quick. In the end, in this case no less than in any other case, there is simply no way to give anybody clear-cut answers. They just have to come up with their own, with their own sense of "*worth*," their own sense of moral cognizance. The realization must finally be that they may never know and may never have a settled sense of what is most worthwhile.

When she returned a year later, Mrs. Albert came bearing gifts for all those who had tried to help: packages of her own chocolate-chip cookies. She had a neatly wrapped package for me, too, when she came to my office. They had eventually decided to go through with an abortion. "That was really hard," she said, "so very hard. I sometimes wonder if I'll ever get over it. It still hurts. I suppose it will always hurt. But, I wanted to tell you that we did get pregnant again, that we now have a beautiful baby, a perfect little boy, just two months old the other day. But it's hard living with what I did, even though I do feel it was the only thing to do, the best of bad choices. I think I'll just love him all the more, knowing that Tommie and I did everything we could to try and save our first. We've grown up an awful lot and are very grateful to the doctors, the nurses, you, and everyone for all you did for us."

Later, after she left and I was munching a cookie, I think I understood what she was trying to say, her need to express gratitude—even more, her sense that we, too, needed to hear it. And I wanted her to know that I, too, was deeply grateful to them for what they helped me learn: it is one thing to understand, quite another to *be understanding,* something she had demonstrated more than once and something I felt would stay with me especially as I continued to try and figure out how truly textured and complicated our moral lives are.

Perhaps, if nothing else—but what could be more important?—this case underscores how critically important it is for people to *talk*, to hear themselves think out loud, and to *be heard,* hoping that they will be able to get through it all with integrity and with the realization that while they might well have acted differently they at least will have a strong sense of having done the very best they could in the circumstances—with all the uncertainty and suffering that entailed.

# SEVEN

# "There I Was, Just Floating . . ."

❖

"You're in medical ethics, aren't you? I remember your name from several things you put into the Hemlock Society's newsletter. I'm a member of it, in fact have been in it for the past eight or nine years."

"'Hemlock?'" I asked. "Yeah, I know the group. Though I'm not a member, I know some people who belong to it. How did you come to join?"

"Well, you know, I know—knew . . . I haven't been very active in recent years—some of the people and, well, I thought that it stood for some good things and just decided to go along and learn what I could. Then when I got really sick a few years later, I really felt bad— my lungs, you know, well they just began to give out—I went to some meetings, read the newsletter more, and so on. What the doctor calls 'emphysema' really took hold. Now, I can hardly go from this chair to the door without giving out, just can't get my breath and have to sit down."

The director of the heart and lung transplant selection committee had asked me to stop by the outpatient clinic to meet Mr. Redstone, who was being evaluated to determine whether he was a suitable candidate for a single-lung transplant. His ex-wife was with him; although divorced, they were still close and she had even agreed to be his main support. The director had asked that I interview all the committee's candidates, not only for lungs but hearts as well. Just what he, or the committee, expected of these discussions was not clear, nor was it clear to me what my own agenda should be. In any event, there I was with Mr. Redstone.

The transplant team's chief pulmonologist had invited me to be there while he went over Mr. Redstone's condition and prospects with and without a transplant and his detailed explanation of what the patient could expect over the next few weeks of evaluation. He also explained what would occur if the patient was accepted as a candidate: the indeterminate waiting period and what would occur once a lung was found, the transplant done, and afterwards.

Dr. Lane's discussion was lucid, full, and frank. Still, Redstone's conduct during the process was curious: he seemed to be so deferential, almost to the point of fawning. His head bobbed up and down and his eyes nervously bounding around the room, only to pounce back to the doctor. His posture was also unusual: slightly hunched over with his elbows resting on his legs while his fingers flitted about weaving and unweaving, his feet tapping a beat on the floor.

After Dr. Lane finished, I was left alone with Mr. Redstone. I explained that I was in ethics and was with him now as part of the transplant team's evaluation process. Although still somewhat nervous, his gesturing and posturing were markedly different, no longer so apparently diffident. Now, instead of his eyes flitting about, he looked straight at me; the inner beat that earlier moved his feet came to a stop; his fingers were no longer quite so busy; he sat up straight; and now he included both his ex-wife and me in his steady gaze. As he had already mentioned the Hemlock Society, I decided to pursue its concerns directly.

"Since you've belonged to Hemlock, Mr. Redstone, I suppose you're familiar with a lot of the issues they talk about?"

"Oh, sure. Sally and I both still belong, and we've discussed those things."

"Great. You've probably already filled out a living will, then.

Have you also talked about the new Durable Power of Attorney for Health Care?"

"Well, actually . . ." the agitated fidgeting returned, "actually, well, you know, well we've talked about all that of course, but, well, you know, actually, I haven't done one of those, those living wills. Neither has Sally . . ."

"Oh? I just figured . . ."

"Well, you know, my doctor, the one I usually see at home, my family doctor . . . the thing is, I did talk to him a few years ago, right after I got so sick, about the living will. He didn't think it was a good idea, he said that he didn't want his hands tied, so I just . . . well I just didn't do one. But you know, I really do believe in that sort of thing."

His ex-wife, Sally, confirmed what the doctor had felt about living wills. "But I don't agree, exactly," she said, "and I haven't gotten around to myself yet."

"Do you know about the new statute, the one the state legislature passed just this year? It became effective last summer, and it does have some new things in it."

"Really? I hadn't realized that," Mr. Redstone replied.

I decided to go straight to the point, rather than take the more indirect route I was inclined to take when I heard their initial reactions. "You know, from what Dr. Lane just told you, you realize that you *do* have a terminal illness; you wouldn't be undergoing evaluation for transplant if it were not terminal."

"I know," he blurted out. "I know, but that's just it, you know? If I can qualify for the lung transplant, then I'm *not* terminal, right? I mean, there's a chance, if a lung gets available, that my disease can be stopped, right?"

"Let's back up a minute, okay? What do you think the living will is all about?"

"Doesn't it say that if you're terminal, the doctors should not do anything? I mean, if you've signed one, it says that you don't want anything done, right? That no life supports, no treatments, should be used."

"Not exactly," I responded. I went on to emphasize a point that I hoped would both explain the point of the living will and would answer his personal physician's misunderstanding of "advance directives," as they've come to be called. "The living will, like the Durable Power of Attorney for Health Care—I'll get back to that in a moment—is one of the ways that people, adults, can indicate what they want to be done whenever they are terminally ill, when their illnesses cannot be reversed and they can longer make their own decisions—when they've lost their decision-making capacity. It's an 'advance directive' that tells physicians what your own wishes would be under those circumstances, when you can no longer tell them yourself. None of this, I realize, is easy to think about. . . ."

"Yeah, I know all that," he replied, "but that's just the point, isn't it? I mean, sure, if nothing can be done about my lungs, well, I'll die sooner or later—probably sooner, from what Dr. Lane said. But, if I'm approved as a candidate for the transplant, then I'm *not* terminal, right? So why sign a living will? Wouldn't it tie Dr. Lane's hands, like my doctor said?"

"Let's back up again, okay? The thing is, this discussion is really important for you and for you, too," I said, including Sally.

"What? Me, too? No one's ever told me that. *Jack's* the one who's sick . . ."

"Right. Not only you, but for your children, too, if they are of legal age. In fact, there's a new federal law, the Patient Self-Determination Act, that becomes effective next December 1 that says in effect that every adult patient entering a hospital or other care facility has certain rights, including the right to refuse treatment, and those facilities have the obligation to inform people of this right, of the right to refuse medical treatment even if they become too sick to speak for themselves. The best way to express this right is to sign a living will and, if you want, a Durable Power of Attorney for Health Care while you are still able to do so. These are the ways in this state that you can express what you want done should you no longer be able to make your own decisions."

"I know that's my right," Mr. Redstone affirmed, "but, again, what if I can get a new lung? Besides, Dr. Lane hasn't said a word about all this." He was becoming a bit agitated.

Clearly no one had talked to him yet or had allowed him to talk about these matters or even thought it appropriate to do so. Probably, I realized, no one on the transplant team wanted to talk, or let him talk, about dying or death. They are, after all, in the business of *saving*, not taking, lives, as they had reminded me on many occasions in the past. In fact, once when I was scheduled to talk at one of the weekly transplant team conferences, I suddenly decided to find out just how much they knew about advance directives and other inherent issues that have come to be called "end-of-life issues." I raised the question before the group and went on to discuss these issues in rather full, somewhat colorful detail—prolonging dying, grief, loss, differences among do-not-resuscitate orders and withdrawal of life supports, withdrawal versus withholding, physician-assisted suicide versus euthanasia. My words fell with a flat thud, and on barren ground.

Thinking back over my faux pas, I remembered that earlier time when I had used that awesome and forbidden word "euthanasia" in that conference about the little boy, Johnny, who was destined for death despite everything that had and could be done. Then, I had faced a stunned silence followed by lively denials. Now I faced just a torpid incomprehension. Nobody wanted to hear any of that stuff, so much so that several of the physicians actively resisted my becoming involved in any way with their patients and, I was later to learn, had actively discouraged any talk about living wills by their patients.

Things began to change, however, when several candidates for transplant openly pointed out to the surgeons and nurses that they had living wills and expected them to be respected. I was called in then to talk about these matters—not, however, with the patients; only with the doctors and nurses. In fact, it was clear to everyone, including the director of the program, that among the matters on the agenda of my discussions with patients and families would be precisely these advance directives and any other end-of-life issues that might be on their minds.

So now, talking with Mr. Redstone and his ex-wife, some square talk was clearly called for. "Several things need to be addressed with both of you. One, you realize—Dr. Lane has already emphasized this—that even if you're accepted as a candidate, a lung might not become available?"

"Sure, we know that. . . ."

"In that event, you realize that you're going to get progressively worse. While you're waiting for a lung, you own lungs will continue to get worse?"

"Sure. . . ."

"Suppose things get so bad that even if a lung becomes available, you might not be in any condition to have it transplanted—what then? What would you want your physicians to do then?"

"If things ever get that bad, I sure don't want them just to keep on plugging away, putting in tubes and such to no end, prolonging the inevitable, you know?"

"Yes, I do understand. But if you've left no clear indication of that, the only thing they *can* do is precisely what you say you *don't want* done. A living will or durable power of attorney for health decisions would prevent that from happening. Moreover, even if a lung is found in time to help you, there is no guarantee, as Dr. Lane emphasized, that it will do the job. You might still be in a condition that can't be treated, that they can't do anything about."

"Lord, Dr. Zaner, it sounds so *awful*, like there's no point in even going on now—you make it all sound so terrible." Sally's despair was wide open.

"That's not my purpose, and I'm truly sorry if I've made you feel badly. It's just that, well, so few people seem willing or able to talk about these matters—like what's actually going on with Mr. Redstone and how he can still retain a good deal of control over what's done and not done for him. Death is no easy matter to discuss at any time, especially with a stranger like myself. Even so, it has to be done; we have to recognize the truth of things, and the truth is that despite everything that the doctors will do for you, if you're accepted—and that is a great deal, for they have a lot at stake here, too, you know—something can go wrong at any time. To deny that, or not talk about it openly, will set you up for some very rough times."

"But . . ." Sally continued, only to be interrupted by him.

"I get his point, Sally, I think. Obviously things can go wrong. A lung might not be found that fits me, or even if they do, it might not work after they put it in, right, doc?"

Now came the really hard part. It was important for him to understand that his condition was terminal. While he did seem aware of that, he also seemed unable to focus on it, to stay there even for a moment; like his hands when the doctor had talked to him earlier, now his mind seemed somehow fluttery and remote, his understanding removed. But that was only the beginning; it seemed to me that from the time when his personal physician had said that he didn't think a living will was needed—it would tie his hands, he had said—Mr. Redstone had just put that sort of thing out of his head. More than that, he had never had more than a sort of glancing thought about his future, his increasingly compromised condition, believing that he was not going to get any better, that he was going to die.

Talking about this in much the same way Dr. Lane had done a few moments earlier, it dawned on me that neither he nor his wife nor many of the doctors he had seen, including his private physician, had actually *read* the living-will document, certainly not the one the state legislature had recently approved. That form makes it very clear that the advance directive to physicians is applicable *only* when the patient is not merely *terminal but also irreversible*, that is, when *all* treatments are futile and nothing else can be done to correct or reverse the terminal condition.

In Mr. Redstone's case, as with any candidate for transplant, while the condition is indeed terminal it is by no means irreversible; that's the hope, the rationale, for placing such patients on the waiting list for a transplant. For that matter, even after a transplant has been done, there is still a considerable chance that it won't work well, or at all; these patients still have, at least for a time, a tenuous hold on life.

Once he understood this, the conversation took on a very different tone, and he quickly saw what I had been driving at: an advance directive is applicable only when he might become so bad off that nothing could help, nothing could rescue him. Then, his physicians would be immensely helped by some indication from him about what to do, what he would want done or not done.

"And," he went directly to what was on his mind, "*up to* that point they won't . . . well, you know, do *less* than what's needed?"

"Of course not," I quickly replied. "Is *that* what's been bothering you?"

"In a way. . . ."

"Charlie," his ex-wife blurted out, "you mean you don't *trust* the doctors?"

"Not exactly," he responded, "but you know, well, it kinda gets to you, you know? I mean, you sign a form that says 'don't treat me any more,' and you have to wonder whether they'll take you seriously, whether that means that when you're really sick, and dying, well, they will just let you go without trying anything else."

"But . . ." I couldn't get my words out before he charged right on.

"I know, it's really silly now that I think it about, see what you're saying. It's not as if people have been worrying about not being treated *enough*; I mean, well, good lord, everything you read is how doctors just won't give up, right? I mean, that's what I came out with from reading a lot of the things from Hemlock, you know?"

This made me think of how so many physicians just don't *talk* with their patients, don't encourage them to discuss what's really on their minds when they are seriously ill, and of how curious that Patient Self-Determination Act is, especially the recent history behind it. Many in health care have recognized that physicians often do not provide for focused discussion to allow the patient the time and presence of mind to think and plan, to retain some control over decisions at the end of life. It was also recognized that it is the doctor's responsibility to encourage this discussion. But what happened? *Hospitals* are required to "inform and educate" patients and families about advance directives; which means, of course, that the onus is put not on physicians but on *patients and families* to ensure that the issue is discussed, most often when they are at the same time experiencing hard times anyway. The hope is, of course, that with more patients understanding their rights to refuse or accept treatments and with greater understanding of the nature of advance directives, more people will be signing them. The hope is also that there will be far more in-depth conversations about these matters in the doctor's office and at the bedside.

In any event, while Mr. Redstone, like other patients, needed some empowerment to think about and insist on this thinking and planning, that was not the only thing on my mind, and I was anxious to get to what seemed to me far more important for him and Sally. I had still not been able to get to the hard part of the conversation.

People being considered for transplants are terminally ill; the purpose of being evaluated medically is to determine in effect whether they are also irreversible; whether they can afford a transplant; whether they have a trustworthy support system to help them through each of the stages of the experience; whether they themselves are compliant and can be trusted to stay with the rigorous personal, medical, and dietary regimen implicit to the entire procedure and for the rest of their lives. In all this, it's not too difficult to see many subtle, complex, and difficult problems that could signify that it is all over for some of these patients unless they can understand and live with what they will have to face for the rest of their lives.

Merely one example made this clear to Mr. Redstone. *If* a single lung is donated; *if* it matches up with his body closely enough; *if* he is then "selected"; *if* he gets through the surgery; *if* things go well in post-surgery; *if* he survives the inevitable rejection and infection episodes; *if* he makes it home and gets to feeling well, he will still have to live with what can only be described at the very best as awkward circumstances. He will have to take powerful medications (immunosuppressants primarily) every day of his remaining life; he will have to return to some medical center for periodic tests to assess the condition of his transplanted organ; and, perhaps most of all, he will have to live with the constant realization that his body could fail him again. In short, he will be "well" *while* having all the signs of "disease"—doctor visits and heavy-duty medications—from then on. He'll be continually reminded by family, friends, acquaintances, employer, and co-workers that he's "not really well."

Mr. Redstone hadn't really thought about all that, nor did he particularly wish to do so now. I, too, thought that enough had been gone over for this session but told him that there were other matters that needed to be discussed to help him and Sally understand the situation far better, especially so that he would understand that getting into this transplant business was and always remains *his choice.* We agreed to meet again the following day in order to give them both a chance to think about matters and then ask questions, raise concerns, or merely listen some more then.

His ex-wife, Sally, was unable to be with us the next day, as she had to be at her office. When Mr. Redstone came into the "quiet room," he seemed very subdued. After exchanging some small talk, I asked whether any questions or concerns had come up overnight. Somewhat haltingly, he began to tell me about a dream, one, he said, that had been occurring rather frequently over the past month or so and that he had had again last night.

"I'm not sure why I'm even telling you this—you're not even a psychiatrist—but, you know, it's really strange, damned strange the more I think about it."

"Why don't you just go ahead and talk about it?"

"I'm just kind of, well, floating around. Not at first, 'cause I'm in bed, you know? Then I hear this siren, like an ambulance, you know? Well, soon as I hear that, I just suddenly am there, with the ambulance. Not with it, but above it, just floating there while the damned thing sounds off, real loud like they do. Then, I just sort of float down right on top of it, and it's all rough and has sharp barbs on it that cut into me. But I can actually see into it, and there's this body there, this guy, who's all bloody and really bad off . . . I can tell, somehow, you know? And, the ambulance folks are there, and working over the guy, trying to stop the blood from pouring out, and the siren is blaring, and they're working, and I'm thinking, 'Wow, I hope his lungs, or at least one of them, is okay.' I could sure use that, you know? But as soon as I begin thinking about that, I get all chilled and cold and don't want to be there. And, as suddenly as I got there, I'm off, floating and feeling real empty . . . real empty. I usually wake up about here and just feel awful. *How could I think that? How could I want this poor guy to die, just so's I can get his lung? That's awful, you know?*"

"You may be right, Mr. Redstone, maybe you should talk this over with someone who knows about dreams and such like. But, you know, what you've said is not all that uncommon. In fact, I'd be surprised if you *didn't* dream or have fantasies like that. Most of the people like you I talk with usually report something like what you've said. Different people, different dreams, in a way, of course, but almost always something that they sense is both disturbing and fascinating, almost like it has you, rather than you having it."

"Yeah, it's really like I can't control things, like it's dreaming me instead of me dreaming it."

As we went on talking about it, about his and other people's "strange" experiences, I tried to get him to focus on several of its dimensions. One thing seemed clear enough, even at first glance: knowing his lungs were rapidly failing, hearing about the possibility of having a transplant and continuing to be alive, and reading about how few people decide to be organ donors (and how few families actually decide to donate the organs of their loved ones). Such patients frequently experience that deeply ambivalent feeling toward other people: wanting *someone* to die so that organs will be donated, yet feeling a profound horror and guilt at that thought. It's one thing to find yourself in a situation where you might feel called on to give your own life for others; it's quite another to be in a condition where you need someone else to die so that you might live. We have a word for the first, "supererogation," actions that are regarded as morally praiseworthy yet are not required of us. We don't have a word when you might be on the receiving end of that, however.

*To give*, we learn from many sources, is a splendid thing; it is at times noble, even divine for some of us. But what of the other side of this? *To receive?* How are you supposed to act when you receive a gift? What ethics govern here? Most of us most of the time think that to receive a gift means we should be grateful in words, possibly in deed, toward the giver. Yet when you really think about it, especially when it's actually happening to you, you know full well that expressions of gratitude can seem so paltry. The more spontaneous the giving and the more precious the gift, the emptier seem our words of thanks. From my experience of talking to people who have been seriously ill who have then become well again, I know immediately what they're going through: words of gratitude just seem to fall so short, seem so inadequate.

What Mr. Redstone seemed to be experiencing was precisely that horror and guilt. He wanted, desperately, not to be where he was, in the need his very body displayed; at the same time, knowing what he needed, he was in the throes of that guilt. But that was hardly the entire story, not the whole theme, behind that dream—even more, behind his troubled feeling. The ambivalence, it seemed to me, concerned not only that but also his having to be on the receiving end of an immensely precious gift—life. And how in the world do you respond to that?

Talking with these patients has made it increasingly apparent that there are many moral issues inherent to what they go through. What I've mentioned is, of course, only several. Ethics has to do in large part with our relationships to other people, how we ought to act toward them. Yet that's not the whole point, for there is always the other side of that, how they ought to act toward us and how we in turn ought to respond to those actions. These relationships themselves can be critical and are surely positive moral facts in their own way.

Potential donors, anonymous as they surely are, are nevertheless experienced by these patients in very complex ways that force difficult moral issues into the open, not the least of which is the troubling realization that these patients will ineluctably be on the receiving end of that profound gift of life that only other people can provide, and then only by dying. Not that they die for us, but merely that they die. But not simply that, either; for this entire "dream" gets going only when others, anonymous others almost always, decide well ahead of time (or their families decide, most often after death) to become "donors," gift-givers for unknown others who need some body part to stay alive. Working with transplant candidates has been a revelation, a rich source of insight into what it means for us to be moral creatures.

# EIGHT

# What Kind of Choice Is That?

❖

I am fascinated by and sometimes leery of much of the research that goes on in many medical centers today, not to mention the remarkable, if also at times exotic, technologies and techniques that come out of it. The human hunger for knowledge is impressive. But it also harbors some hard ethical, economic, political, and social problems. To understand the nature of these issues, especially the wholly novel moral problems that are implicit to the new developments in genetics, some understanding of human genetics is unavoidable. This was dramatically brought home to me when I was asked to become involved in several cases.

For instance, several years ago David Johnson, a physician specializing in genetics, stopped me as I made my way to the hospital from my office. He wanted to know what I thought about a problem that had just come up. It seems that the gene that causes cystic fibrosis (CF) had been recently located. Moreover, the techniques used in the discovery were also, in effect, tests that detect whether any individual, from fetuses to adults, carries the gene. This test was first used in sperm banks, donor sperm being part of artificial insemination (AI) programs available to infertile couples seeking pregnancy.

"We're one of several centers where batches of donated sperm are being tested for CF," Dr. Johnson told me.

"Really? That's really putting the foot to the floor, isn't it? I mean, the gene was only just discovered, and already there's a test."

"Of course," he replied. "If we can prevent people using AI from getting sperm carrying the CF gene, that's a real service. Anyway, we began doing the test recently and, wouldn't you know it, we found a positive batch. The first one tested in any center to turn up positive."

"What are you doing about it?"

"Well, that's why I stopped you. As it turns out, sperm from this batch has already been used for AI, and there have been four successful pregnancies."

His words sort of hung in the air. My thoughts did too, as the import of his words began to sink in. "You mean . . ."

"Yep. To make things even more difficult, one baby was already born two months ago. Another is well on its way and should be born in about a month or so, as the pregnancy is between thirty-two and thirty-three weeks gestation. The other two are less far along. If everything goes okay they won't be delivered for about six months. They are about twelve or thirteen weeks along. The question is what do we do about these cases? The options are limited for the parents of the second one, as therapeutic abortion can't be offered, but we can offer it to the parents of the last two fetuses."

"Has the donor of the sperm been informed? That seems to me the first thing you should think about."

"Well, we've already done that."

"Did he agree to be told? I mean, there'd be a problem if he was asked and didn't want to know."

"Fortunately, that wasn't a problem. I agree, though, that we'd be in a bit of a bind if he'd refused the test. After all, if he ever tried to donate again we'd have to refuse to accept his sperm, and then he'd know anyway. I don't know what we'd do, though, if we found out that he went elsewhere to donate sperm. Most places are testing for genetic disorders now, but some aren't."

"That'd be a real problem, of course. But what about confidentiality? I mean, if it should become known that he's a CF carrier, there's a real chance that he could become . . ."

"Stigmatized? Yeah, we've been concerned about that, but I think we've got that under control. All the donors are kept strictly anonymous."

"I realize that, Dave, but it might be wise to take some extra precautions."

"I agree; that should be on our agenda, too, when we meet. Right now, though, it's another set of problems we've got that I'd like you to think about: the couples who got samples of that batch of sperm."

"Well, if I get what you're asking, don't you have to inform them, too? Even more, you've got to bring them all in and ask about testing, right? Especially the couple whose baby is already born. You need to let them know what happened."

"Sure, but to be effective we need to test the mother, since her egg was used in the procedure. You know about cystic fibrosis, don't you?"

"Maybe you'd better tell me, Dave, so I can get a better idea of what's at stake."

"Why don't I just give you some materials that will explain all about it, then when you've gone through them, call me and we'll get a group together to see where we stand."

Cystic fibrosis is a genetic disease. Like all of these diseases, it isn't contagious like infectious diseases. In fact some of them may lie dormant for years, even generations, before symptoms appear. While genetic-based diagnosis may be used to confirm an underlying condition, it is most often celebrated for its ability to detect and predict future disease for persons who are not currently sick or disabled.

A baby gets CF from its parents who, until the discovery of the gene, often didn't and couldn't know that they had passed the disease to their baby. CF is *autosomal recessive*: the baby can't get the disease unless it is carried by both parents, and then there is only a one in four chance that the baby will have CF and a two in four chance that the baby will itself be a carrier. The genetic test thus determines if parents are carriers, are persons who have one "CF-causing" gene and one "CF-preventing" gene. Carriers do not have the disease and have no personal health problems from having only one CF-causing gene. Overall, about four in one hundred Caucasians in the United States are carriers; the statistics are much less for other races. Since both parents must be carriers for the baby to have that 25-percent chance of getting CF, if only one parent is a carrier the children almost never have the disease, though some could be carriers.

Cystic fibrosis causes thick mucus to form in the lungs, making the individual cough, and leads to lung damage over time. They are often sick with lung infections and may need to be hospitalized. It also causes poor digestion of food, and for this reason children with CF may have problems growing and gaining weight. Unhappily, although the discovery of the CF-causing gene made the genetic test possible, there is currently no cure. Still, medicines and therapies have been developed that help people with CF feel better and live longer—though treatment can take a lot of time each day and is expensive. Some children with CF die very young, but most now live to be adults, usually dying before they are forty. Things are getting much better, however: in 1970, only half of all children with CF lived past fourteen; now half live to be about twenty-eight.

To know whether the baby from that first AI pregnancy had a chance of being born with full-blown CF, it was necessary to test the fetus, or at least the mother. In either case, of course, the mother couldn't be avoided; she would have to give consent in either case. All that was known was that the "father," the donor of the sperm, tested positive as a carrier. If the mother also tested carrier-positive, then the baby's chances of having CF would go up substantially. If the mother tested negative the baby could be no more than a carrier. If it were important to know if the baby was a carrier, then it could be tested much later.

I didn't see any particular problems about discussing the matter with the mother and her husband. She should certainly be told, right?

But as I read through more of the literature Dr. Johnson had given me, I began to realize at least one potential problem. A lot of people refuse to have genetic tests done. They just don't want to know. The "right of self-determination," as we've come to call this, does in fact include the right to refuse medical advice and treatment, including diagnostic tests. Suppose she refused the test? That's her choice. But things could get sticky if her husband *did* want to know.

As mentioned earlier, the second pregnancy was too far along, ruling out a therapeutic abortion whether or not tests proved positive for mother and then fetus. As in the first case, though, she should surely be offered the test for herself and for her fetus. If she tested positive, the baby had a 25-percent chance of actually having CF and a 50-percent chance of being a carrier. Suppose the dice fell badly, both she and her fetus test positive? The couple would then at least have some time to prepare themselves, make appropriate contacts with physicians knowledgeable about CF, and even begin setting aside money to help pay for future care. Still, that's a pretty awful future to know about in advance.

But it seemed to me that the last two pregnancies harbored issues that were even more complicated and potentially explosive. If the parents, one or both, refused the test, there was still a chance that their babies would have CF or would be carriers, thus potentially placing them and their offspring at some risk of the disease. Of course, if either of the mothers themselves tested positive, then even without the prenatal test of the fetuses they would know that their developing babies had that 25-percent chance of having CF, or a 50-percent chance of being carriers. Whatever was done or not done, these parents faced the difficulties and suffering of making decisions based on information that could only be uncertain and chancy. Only if the parents agreed to have the developing fetuses tested and the tests turned up positive would they know that these future babies would suffer all the problems of cystic fibrosis. While the test isn't perfect, it is very highly reliable. With a positive result, they could, and most surely would, be offered the option of therapeutic abortion, as both fetuses were still in the first trimester.

Here we enter more difficult moral terrain. Beyond the problems that had already emerged, there is also the fact that all these couples went to some lengths to have a baby. They *chose* to have children by going through with artificial insemination. Thus, even to suggest abortion to such couples could well open up some serious issues. The deliberate choice, the attempts at adoption, then AI all strongly indicate that such parents will likely be deeply against that step, and if they chose abortion they could well suffer seriously in years to come.

Many parents are opposed to therapeutic abortion even under normal circumstances. But are these circumstances "normal"? Is it right to refuse abortion when you *know* that the baby will have CF? Is it right to *force* a baby to live with this disease when you have it in your power to prevent this from happening? Since there are currently no ways of stopping the ravages of cystic fibrosis, no magic bullets that could prevent it while the baby is still in the womb (or for that matter after birth), "preventing it from happening" *means* abortion. But what kind of "choice" is this, especially if choosing abortion means violating a basic moral concern?

On the other hand, many people are *not* opposed to abortion, especially in light of this sort of genetic knowledge. Some of these people are women who are currently pregnant. They would doubtless choose abortion for genetic reasons, and who can fault them? No matter what a parent's position on abortion, babies are the future, and some of them will also become parents, passing on genetic traits to their children and their children's children. There is no evading this awesome set of questions. The new genetic knowledge opens up wholly new areas of control, or it at least allows physicians (and those who supply funding to them) to exercise serious influence over the things that are known. This in turn puts new choices in their hands. Knowing that a fetus has or carries a genetic disease *means* that we can now act to influence or change the course of events. We can choose to stop that life in its tracks, and, if carried out as a general policy, we can choose to stop genetic disease in its tracks. But choice and action unavoidably carry moral responsibility for what is chosen and acted upon.

Whatever the parents of the last two fetuses at risk for CF decide to do, to abort or not to abort, they have unavoidably made a moral choice. They will have acted in the light of what they know and must not only live with the consequences but also bear the responsibility of their choice. In these circumstances, choosing not only affects this particular fetus, but future ones as well. There's no way around it. A really different sort of moral concern has emerged. Thanks to genetic discoveries and the tests they make possible, we have become increasingly responsible in a very direct way for future generations.

All this became painfully apparent when I was asked to consult in another case involving all of these issues. Meet Mary and Jim Blackman: Mary and Jim met at college, where she majored in biology and he in business. They both had jobs they enjoyed. She had planned on going on to medical school, but put that on hold when they decided to get married. They both wanted children, and she became pregnant several years later. She hadn't realized (and apparently he didn't know this either) that she had married into a family at risk for genetic disease. Several members of Jim's family lived close by, and there were regular visits and family talk. She began to suspect that something was going on when she learned that his grandfather, an uncle, and a cousin had all died under what seemed unusual circumstances, and nobody was willing to talk much about them. She suspected something genetic, but family members were not helpful. For a time, she was left having to wonder.

By the time I got involved, her suspicions about Jim's family had peaked. An inherited faulty gene that results in a rare and lethal disease, Huntington's chorea, was apparently being passed on from parent to child, "segregating," in his extended family, the "kindred." Huntington's is a rare hereditary disease characterized by a wide variety of rapid, highly complex, and jerky movements, "chorea," that appear well coordinated but in fact are involuntary because that gene has ceased to work properly. Chronic and progressive, this disease has a variable age of onset, but it most often occurs at about forty years of age and results in mental deterioration, dementia, and death within ten to fifteen years.

Unlike cystic fibrosis, Huntington's is known to be caused by a single gene. Shortly before I got involved with the Blackmans, a test for the disease had been somewhat fortuitously discovered. Studying a relatively closed society in Venezuela, most of whose members had Huntington's, a "genetic marker" or "linkage," the G-8 probe, had been identified. Like many genetic discoveries, the linkage showed that Huntington's was segregating in that Venezuelan kindred. Researchers found a tiny piece of DNA, which carries the genetic code for each human being, that apparently travels along or is linked with the defective gene. Although it doesn't test for the gene itself, the linkage is 95 to 98 percent accurate; the linking segment of DNA is almost always found in people who have the disease. With this probe, it can thus be rather accurately determined whether an individual carries the gene well before any symptoms appear; in fact, it can be done prenatally, as early as eight or ten weeks into a pregnancy. As a linkage test, it must be done on large numbers of people to determine just which specific segment of DNA is linked with the gene for each family or kindred tested. Tests with that kindred in Venezuela, of course, confirmed that Huntington's is transmitted as an *autosomal dominant* trait: only one parent needs to carry the faulty gene to be affected and to pass it on to children, each of whom has a 50-percent chance of getting it. The parent need not be symptomatic in order to pass it on. Indeed, most are not. Children are most often born before the parent is forty, which indicates one of the harsh difficulties connected with this genetic flaw. A child can receive the gene and neither the parent nor the child know of its presence. The transmitting parent may not even know that he or she is a carrier. At some point the symptoms begin showing, followed by a gradual decline to incapacity and death. When symptoms first appear, they only know that something is terribly wrong.

I had learned about the G-8 probe in the newspaper item. Mrs. Blackman, still having the dream of becoming a physician, had been in the habit of reading medical journals and had learned about the probe shortly before the news hit the public media. She had immediately asked her obstetrician about it to see whether she and her fetus could be tested. The obstetrician had not yet heard of the discovery, much less that a test was available. She gave him a copy of the medical report and requested another visit in the near future. They knew that she was about twelve weeks pregnant, and she was anxious to have the option of abortion if her developing fetus were tested and found to be positive. Her anxiety was obvious. She promptly talked to her husband about his family history. She even asked him to have the test and to agree to have the fetus tested. She then proceeded to ask about family members' being tested. Since the test is for linkage, not for the gene itself, and these linkages vary somewhat from family to family, she realized that the most accurate results would require that others in his family also agreed to be tested.

Mr. Blackman refused to discuss the matter with her and bawled her out for bringing his family into the picture. He simply didn't want to know or hear any more about the matter. He didn't want her bothering the family, either. She asked several family members anyway but couldn't find any of them willing to talk about it much less agree to be tested. Such refusals are not surprising. Studies have shown that about a third of the people at risk for Huntington's do not want to know. Even one of the co-discoverers of the G-8 probe did not want to have the test done, although she was at risk for the disease and knew it was segregating in her own immediate and extended family.

Mrs. Blackman felt it was deeply unfair to bring a child into the world with that awful disease ahead of it and with the chance of passing it on to its children's children. What should she do? When we later met, she told me that when she returned to her doctor he had read about the probe. He also told her that the genetics unit at the regional medical center could perform the prenatal test. As they discussed the matter, it became obvious to both of them that if she were to have the prenatal test and learn that her baby were affected, she would then know that her husband had the gene. He was not yet showing any symptoms, but with no treatments at hand, nothing could be done for him when he did, as he surely would. In spite of this, if the baby tested positive, she felt she would *have* to tell her husband, for she knew she would choose to abort. If she didn't tell him and had the abortion anyway, he would then surely know about himself whether she told him or not and whether he wanted to hear it or not. Her dilemma was excruciating. It seemed as though her world was crumbling even though she as yet knew nothing.

It was at this point that her obstetrician referred her to our center. She had decided to see a specialist in prenatal diagnosis at the center and, not knowing exactly how to handle it, he asked me to help out. A meeting with her was arranged. During our conversation, she told me what had gone on before. She struck me as highly intelligent, caring, sensitive, and shattered.

"We really want a baby," she said in an emotionally charged voice, "but I just can't go through with it, not with *this* hanging over us. But Jim just refuses, just doesn't want to know."

"I gather you've told him about the baby's future, if it's affected?"

"Sure, but he acts like he doesn't hear me. He just gets angry, tells me to shut up and leave well enough alone. 'Well enough!' My God, how can *anyone* say that forcing a baby to live with Huntington's is 'leaving well enough alone'? It's not *right* for him to refuse, is it?"

"But you don't yet know that your baby is affected, do you?"

"Not yet, but from what I've seen, I already know that four or five people in Jim's family *must* have had Huntington's. They had all the symptoms, and there's just no way they could have died like they did in any other way. I've been reading everything I can get my hands on since I read about that probe."

"But you can't be sure . . ."

"I know that, but there's a way now that I can be almost certain, and I just can't get it through that thick head of his . . ."

"Is there any chance your husband would be willing to come in to talk about things with me?"

"I've tried and tried, but he just refuses, and now he's become so *firm*. And that's just *wrong*. Nobody else in the family will discuss it, either; they're all just as pig-headed as he is. Maybe that's a genetic trait, too! But it's just so wrong to risk our baby like that, isn't it?"

Obviously, there were no easy answers to her dilemma. It was clear, though, that she was determined to have the test done. She knew that even if the test were negative there was still a chance it was mistaken and if it were positive, it could also be mistaken, though the chances of either a false negative or a false positive were very slight. She was already convinced, though, that the baby was affected and that was quite enough. What she really wanted at this point was confirmation.

All I could advise was that she keep trying to get her husband to agree, if not to being tested then at least to her having it done on her fetus. Then, if the test were positive, she should try her best to get him to come in for serious counseling, since he would then know full well what was in store for him and counseling would be urgent for both of them. He was only twenty-eight years old; while he still had probably ten or so years of unsymptomatic life ahead, he could still be helped to understand and make some plans.

It was obvious that she had already decided to have the test. In fact, she was scheduled the next day. I urged her to wait a few days, since the way things were going a split between them seemed almost inevitable. What eventually happened realized her worst nightmare: the baby tested positive, and her husband still adamantly refused to discuss matters, much less be tested or come in for counseling. She decided to proceed with abortion anyway. Inevitably, when he learned about it there was a terrible scene. They were divorced shortly afterwards. Since he continued to refuse counseling and she moved out of state, I never learned what happened to either of them.

The dilemmas associated with these genetic diagnoses are awesome. Matters are complicated by the fact that while the new genetic research provides profound information, there are few if any treatments. Still, research is moving ahead rapidly and looking into ways of correcting or at least slowing the progression of these diseases. But until some way of curing, correcting, or slowing is at hand, can any of us blame a person for refusing to take a genetic test, or for not wanting to know results if it is done, when a virtual death sentence is the basic message and nothing can then be done about it?

The information is so devastating, as I learned from the Blackmans, that one even wonders whether without effective therapies the results of such tests should be made available at all to those tested. In the absence of treatments, the bearers of bad news, the physicians and researchers, may be subject to severe criticism, even condemnation, like modern-day Cassandras. On the other hand, the refusal to be tested and informed merely passes the problem on to a different set of persons—spouses and children in the kindred, present and future—who are then confronted with the very same dilemmas. Is that morally right? The individual's treasured privacy and freedom of choice seem somehow dubious in the light of what is passed on to others and the responsibility that choice invariably carries with it.

By choosing abortion, Mrs. Blackman tried to save their child from later having to face an agonizing decision about bearing offspring; if she had chosen not to abort, they would have still chosen for their child, who must then live with the disease and must face the same agonizing choice of whether to save its children from that very same decision. Only by abortion, apparently, can these agonizing decisions be stopped. However, by preventing the very *existence* of a child at all, they will have foreclosed the possibility of its exercising its own freedom of choice. While an individual like Mr. Blackman is only exercising *his* right of self-determination, those other people, children present and future, are thereby denied that same right. A person who is unwilling to confront issues having direct bearing on family and offspring *determines* that a future of terrible suffering will be *passed on*. In either case, their future is determined without their having had any choice in the matter. Should the exercise of *our* freedom cancel our children's equally justified right to *their* freedom?

Raising that difficult issue only serves to make another cluster of enigmas crop up. To know about her fetus's genetic traits, it was necessary to find out about the genetic codes of Mr. Blackman's family and kindred. In light of this, consider the pressures that could readily be brought on those people, many of whom she had never met and about whom she knew next to nothing. Beyond the Blackman's, if we think about how fragmented the family has become in our times it's easy to appreciate the difficulty of tracing out genetic lines in our society.

Consider, too, that given the way many genetically transmitted diseases show up in as-yet unsuspecting relatives, the pressures for genetic testing could well attract the interests of insurance companies, employers, and still others. None of these parties has been particularly shy about trying to gain access to such information and making use of it. Think about AIDS, for instance. Confidentiality could well become little more than a sort of nostalgic relic, if it isn't already, and the control of this potent information poses critical social issues. When you add in the long-term costs of illness, the considerable expense of diagnostic tests, not to mention the medical and hospital costs of care connected with these diseases, things can quickly get even more out of hand than they are already in this time of scarce resources and funds. Does society have a right to invoke prepayment, taxation, or other schemes to offset the inevitable cost of these diseases? If it makes sense to call for health care for everyone, does this include even those at risk for passing on genetic diseases? Should it include people who, like Mr. Blackman, will at some point come down with a genetic disease? The health care system is already heavily burdened. If nothing else breaks the system, adding these costs may well do just that.

All of these issues plagued me as I was grappling with the problems presented by the Blackmans. Do we really have an *individual* "right of choice" when a refusal to be tested places countless *other* people at serious risk? Does "informed consent" apply to an individual when critical information about others in an individual's family and kindred is needed in order to know whether babies (present and future) might be afflicted with a devastating genetic disease and thus end up passing it on to other generations? Do we as a society have an obligation to "clean up the gene pool," as geneticists express it? What would this do to our cherished value of self-determination? "All persons are born equal" is just not true, not literally. We are obviously *not equal* in numerous ways, including our biological wherewithal and genetic inheritance. We also differ in our familial circumstances, racial and ethnic sources, personal histories and talents, life-styles, and still other ways. *Should* any of these differences *make a difference*—morally, economically, politically, socially? If so, what is that difference? We haven't done very well in the recent or distant past in equalizing such differences as job opportunity or education. Is there any reason to expect we'll do any better now when we must add our genetic endowments to that list of differences? In our history, unless there is a clear threat to the common good, individual rights have taken priority over the social good. Often this has worked for us. What about now? The new genetics challenges our deeply embedded sense of priority, free choice, privacy, and informed consent.

I once heard a geneticist express an aspect of the difficulty: "People who belong to a kindred where a serious disorder is segregating have a moral obligation to permit information to be kept in registers." She went on to argue that we are obligated even to submit to genetic tests as they become available. This came to mind while I was talking with Mrs. Blackman, and I had to wonder whether this applied to her. Would this moral obligation apply to Mr. Blackman? Should he have submitted to finding out what he freely chose *not* to know? Does the good of others—especially his own developing baby—take precedence over his right to choose for himself? Suppose, despite every effort to respect his privacy, it became known that he has Huntington's: who has a right to that information? Does his employer? His insurance agency? How can that information be kept private?

Many geneticists think that when the suffering of other people can be prevented, our moral priorities must be changed. I've heard it said, for instance, that the very idea of "privacy" may have to be altered if one person's insistence on not entering a register could indirectly cause suffering to other persons. If that is correct, did Mr. Blackman have a greater *obligation* to be tested than a right to exercise his freedom of choice since his own baby was at risk? If he himself were positive, what would happen to his child when he becomes symptomatic, demented, and then dies? Surely that awful kind of suffering should be prevented if at all possible.

Whether you agree or disagree with these geneticists, you can't escape the critical problems posed by their discoveries, many more of which are being announced almost daily, as we now realize. Our moral traditions do not help much to resolve these problems; indeed, they in some part create the difficulties. After all, it was not only that couple's own baby who was at risk. If nothing were done and nothing learned about it, and the husband and baby were indeed tested positive for Huntington's, not only would that baby and its father come to suffer that devastating disease but the baby would soon be deprived of a father. If the child were born and later had children, they too would have that 50-percent chance of inheritance, as would their children and on and on. People *now alive* as well as innumerable *future generations* will be condemned to suffer.

While our moral traditions counsel us to respect other people as individuals and grant them what we enjoy, the freedom to choose, we are also counseled not to harm other people—the Golden Rule. But this rule has always been thought to apply only to neighbors, to other people who are *present*; we are only responsible in various ways to those living *at the same time* as we do. The Blackmans' dilemma forced me to realize that the new genetics has made that limited connection somehow not enough. Being able not only to know crucial things about their genetic makeup, but also to change things— whether through abortion, birth control, or the newly developing gene-splicing techniques—our moral responsibilities extend to future generations. How can we know, though, what's "best" for them? Are *our* current values so supreme that they would be endorsed without question by people in the future? Obviously, to know that requires far more wisdom than any of us has or even believes possible. As one of my teachers, Hans Jonas, once said, "we need wisdom most when we believe in it the least!" *Is* there such wisdom?

Future generations have become part of our moral ambiance. Traditional moral insight has counseled obligations first and foremost to those most immediate to us: our families, our friends, our neighbors. To some extent, to be sure, parts of these traditions sought to remind us of our duties to strangers, even to our enemies. This emphasis, however, does not concern future generations, and thus seems but a relic in the hectic, aggressive, technological societies of the twentieth century. Appeals to our traditions just won't do now. For genetic testing and consequent knowledge to be truly useful, entire families and kindreds must agree to be tested. If any refuse, they may well thereby cause harm to other people. Others may suffer, not from the sort of direct harmful actions our moral traditions have rightly condemned, but from the exercise of precisely one of our most cherished convictions: personal choice to refuse tests and treatments.

Abortion has made us aware of something like this complexity. But isn't one of the reasons it has caused such dispute and violence exactly that our usual moral insights don't help, that we have to come to the point of literal violence precisely *from* our respective moral beliefs? This may well harbor one of the most significant moral issue of our times: violence, whether verbal or physical, and, on the other hand, its moral opposite, tolerance. Are there honest and humane ways of resolving the issues that so deeply divide us today? We all know how so many arguments are provoked, often by the slightest itch or look, and how these arguments go on interminably and rarely, if ever, result in anything like compromise or negotiated settlement. Perhaps there is no settling such disputes, for neither basic starting-point—"life is sacred" or "right of choice"—seems commensurable with the other. Nothing short of starting from some other premise, which most of those most committed to the arguments seem unwilling to consider, seems capable of anything like a resolution. Can we any longer truly tolerate differences?

With the new genetics, matters threaten to get even more out of hand. Unquestionably, trying to ameliorate the ravages of genetic disease is a noble and worthwhile aim. Who doesn't keenly feel the outrageous, utterly unjust misfortune visited on the unwitting victims of Huntington's, cystic fibrosis, muscular dystrophy, Hurler's, or any of the several thousand genetic diseases already known? On the other hand, can any of us really know with any certainty how to answer that desperate pregnant woman's urgent questions?

As if these issues were not enough, the curative aims of the new genetics are not the only thing on the new moral agenda. If genetics is capable of gene splicing, gene surgery, and gene therapy and yields knowledge of how to correct genetic flaws, it also provides the kind of knowledge that can be used for quite different purposes. Along with the therapeutic promise is the *eugenic* potential to alter the subtle cellular messages in our genes and chromosomes so as to alter the what and who of those who inherit them—our children, and their children's children. Just as breeds of cattle can and have been "improved," so, too, are blueprints at hand for "improving" human kind, whether it be our memories, our physiques, or the balance of the sexes. To "improve," however, implies not just the knowledge of *how* to go about doing it; it also implies the *wisdom* to know what, how, and, most of all, *whether* it should be done at all, to know which ends or goals are preferable, which are worthy. Can any of us be entrusted with that?

Mrs. Blackman's conviction, painful though it surely was, is instructive even though insufficient. With these genetic tests, we witness a change in the very sense of what we understand by "moral agent": the single, isolated individual, her husband. Rather, the new moral agent is something somehow larger, more complex: both she and her husband and their developing fetus, *all together*. Yet, not even that is sufficient. For at stake is also his brothers and sisters, who need to know as much as he does and for their children's sakes. Even more, there are his first and second and third cousins—the entire kindred, and for all those same reasons. For that matter, there are all those future people, their children, and on and on.

There has appeared on the scene a different sort of moral fact, one that has perhaps been around without our realizing it, or having to realize it, and much of the centering core of our traditional moral thinking simply isn't capable of working with that new moral fact. It seems that individuals *must* now, if not all along, be considered only *in relation to and in relationship with* other individuals who at the very least share the same or similar genetic endowments and histories.

Mrs. Blackman described her husband as acting *immorally* when he exercised his otherwise well-justified right of free choice in refusing. Doing so, his baby, himself, his wife were put at risk by his deliberate choice. *Taken in context*, to be moral, she thought, *he really had no choice.* Every individual person is related in complex and morally significant ways to certain other persons, and *these relationships themselves carry moral weight*—in situations like hers, *decisive* weight.

We are connected to other people through friendships, love, associations, affiliations, and, more broadly as a culture and people, shared histories. These connections can be ignored only at our moral peril, just the sort of peril that woman experienced so deeply, and doubtless her husband as well, in his own way, at the time and later, after the abortion and divorce. I don't think that her conviction and what she helped me understand mean that rethinking our moral lives requires us to give priority to society; that, from what we know in our own century, would be intolerable. The point is, rather, that we have to rethink our moral traditions, not only individualism and its moral consequences, but beyond that the usual way of pitting the individual against society. That opposition can't be right, either. What we need is a different way of thinking about what is good, right, and fair, and we need to appreciate how our promising discoveries place us willy-nilly in the embrace of wholly new choices and new forms of responsibility. And we need, in the end, to learn what to make of the differences among us, whether they shall divide us with violence or bring us together in tolerance, split us into aggressive factions or unite us in our common humanity.

# N I N E

# "That Damned Machine . . ."

❖

A tall, sinewy man in his late thirties, Joe Blanton worked at an auto-parts company and helped out part-time at the small town's fire department. He was not married, though he did have a girlfriend. When I met him much later, he related his story to me. While he was at the auto-parts store, he said that he "all of a sudden" got hot and nauseous and had to go to the bathroom and vomit. Several of his co-workers noted that he "looked really bad." They urged him to get to the hospital, but he didn't feel like that was necessary.

He continued to feel "really awful" and later in the day decided that he'd better go find out what was wrong. He called his family doctor, who agreed to meet him at the local hospital. When he arrived, his doctor ran some tests and, almost immediately, Mr. Blanton was told that he had a kidney problem. As there were still some things that were unclear, however, he was advised to stay in the hospital. He told me that he stayed there for three days while other tests were run. As his doctor, a general practitioner, was still somewhat unclear about what was going on, he was advised to go to the regional medical center to see a specialist. And there we eventually met.

"That was a great hospital," Mr. Blanton noted sarcastically. "All they did was take urine specimens. On the third day I was there they did a biopsy, then sent me home. Great! They never did tell me anything, about a diet or nothing, except that I had something wrong with my kidneys. They said they'd have to wait on the biopsy, then I would have to go back."

Meanwhile, his feet began to swell and he got "really tired" even walking across the room. His family doctor said his difficulty breathing was because he had a sinus problem. He became very concerned about his job; his feet and face continued to swell, and he was not getting any answers from his doctor. He finally got to the point where he couldn't breathe at all well, so he went to the local hospital's emergency room. He was told that he was hyperventilating.

"At the time, my lungs were full of liquid; the doc there didn't know it and I didn't know it, but I *wasn't* hyperventilating."

Still very worried about his job at the auto-parts store, he eventually let them know that he would just have to take some time off. They agreed. At about the same time, he was scheduled to attend a class in firefighting, which he was required to take or lose that job. Since he had already told the auto-parts place that he couldn't work for a while, he felt he just had to keep up the requirements of the firefighting position. But, he said, "I couldn't breathe, walk, or move around much. And I couldn't see. When I walked out of the house, everything had 'snow' on it. It was unbelievable." He managed, though, to attend the class.

Several weeks after the biopsy had been done, he still had heard nothing and decided to return to the local hospital to try and find out what was going on. The biopsy report had just come in from the lab and was suggestive of serious renal problems. In addition, his blood count and hemoglobin were very low. He was told that he should return immediately to the medical center and was promptly whisked off in an ambulance. There, he told me, everything happened "way too fast: just click, click, click." A catheter was placed in his arm, and he was promptly "hooked up to a kidney machine, which I'd never heard of before." While he was being dialyzed, Mr. Blanton related to me, he was "kinda surprised because all of my family was up there, you know, and when you see everybody you haven't seen for ten or eleven years, you think, 'Well, this is it. I'm a goner.'"

While he was being brought to the medical center, his mother, two brothers, sister, several aunts and uncles, and three cousins had been told by his family doctor that he "probably didn't have much of chance to make it" but that the doctors at the medical center would make every effort to keep him alive. His mother was jolted. The family doctor had even told *him* that there wasn't much of a chance but that they were going to try. "Anyway," he said, "I woke up on the machine and all the folks were right there! That kind of scared me. I thought for sure that it was all over. I mean, it looked like a wake, you know? 'Course, I know now that it wasn't all that bad."

Probably because of the crowd of people around him and their anxiety, the nurse taking care of him at the time became concerned. She decided to page me. A short time after she beeped me and got no response, she decided that things were threatening to boil over—his mother and several others there were very upset—and called me at home, demonstrating again what being "on call" means. After listening to her, I called the attending physician and related what she had said. Apparently, she had already talked to him, as he quickly agreed that it would be good to have me involved. He emphasized, too, that he had talked with the family and had tried to straighten things out. He wasn't sure, though, that they believed him. I immediately went to the hospital.

It was obvious which room he was in, as the hubbub carried rather far out into the halls. I went in, introduced myself to the group, and explained that Mr. Blanton's physician thought that I might be able to help. I was promptly assailed with questions, which I managed to duck while I moved over to his bed. He was fairly alert and clearly agitated.

"Mr. Blanton . . ." I began.

"Who are you? I mean, what's going on here? Are you *another* of them damned doctors? What's going on?"

Questions from the family kept drumming in, so I decided that a direct approach was needed. "If you all will be still a moment; all the racket is not helping Mr. Blanton, and I can't get all the questions anyway. Mr. Blanton," I turned directly to him, "are you able to talk?"

"Hell, yes, nothin's wrong with that. I mean, I don't feel very good about this damned machine, but what the hell, I still can hear and think."

"Well, Dr. Case asked me to try to help get things clear with everyone. I understand that there was some confusion about what's happening to you?"

"Damned straight," he pounced on the opening. "Ol' Doc Smithers back home told everyone, even me, that I was goin' to die."

"But, your doctor here, Dr. Case, *has* clarified all that, hasn't he?"

"Oh, yeah, no problem about that. I mean, don't I feel fine now? Hell, yes, but I know my kidneys, well, they've just sorta quit, all of a sudden-like. You know? And, I gotta be on this damned machine, at least until I can get a new one."

"Great, then you and," I turned to the crowd, "all of you do understand that he is not going to die—I mean, not right now? You understand that he needed dialysis badly, and now that he's getting his blood cleaned out he'll be okay?"

Obviously, Dr. Case had done a great job with this family; though they were peeved at Dr. Smithers, they did seem to understand things and were apparently clear about what was going on now. We talked for a time, as, from what Dr. Case had picked up, it was important that everyone there clearly understand the patient's actual condition: that end-stage renal disease (ESRD) is a serious matter, that dialysis would of course help, and that a renal transplant should certainly be given much thought. For the moment, though, I thought it more important just to let them air their concerns and for me to listen.

It became clear that Mr. Blanton was deeply concerned about what all this and a transplant would cost. Although he had several jobs, he did not have much insurance and, for the moment, was worried that he just wouldn't be able to pay for "all that stuff."

"I have to pay the bills, you know? At least, 80 percent of them; the government's supposed to pay the rest. That's what that social worker said. But, I can't even pay what's left over. We are poor folks. Don't have that kind of money. Sure, I'm a veteran, and they're supposed to take care of people like us over at the VA, right? And they pay for everything. At least, that's what the lady said."

As if he hadn't thought about it before, right then and there he decided he had to transfer to the VA hospital, even though he was told that he stood a better chance for a transplant if he stayed where he was. He felt he had to go the VA, though, because "everything is paid for there, you know."

Apparently, the rush to the hospital was not particularly necessary after all, or so I thought at the time. After he had transferred to the VA I got a call from Dr. Case. He had been called by the specialist at the VA, who told him that one of his patients, Mr. Joe Blanton, had been asking whether he couldn't see me. His attending physician at the VA, Dr. Reviso, didn't know me, so he'd called Dr. Case, whom he knew had taken care of Mr. Blanton a short time at the medical center. I told Dr. Case that I probably couldn't do anything as long as the patient was in the VA hospital. The VA system had yet to recognize clinical ethics as such, and I hadn't been involved in patient-care issues there. In any event, I decided to call Dr. Reviso at the VA to find out why Mr. Blanton had asked about seeing me. As it turned out, he just wanted to talk, which seemed okay to me and the VA; they just considered me like any visitor. I managed to see him several times during the next week, during which time the full story came out.

Twice a week for the next eight weeks, he drove to the VA for dialysis. He then managed to get a dialysis machine at home, furnished by the VA, where he continued dialysis three times a week and "don't pay for a thing." Unable to work all this time, he had applied for Social Security. "I get disability from them but it hasn't started yet. It's been months. They keep telling me it will come through, just give it time. I told the lady, though, that they were about to repossess everything I have, which they are. It's been three months and if you can't make a payment, the people kinda want their money. They don't seem to care about what I'm goin' through, and my mom sure can't help out. She doesn't have that kind of money, either. Neither does anybody else in the family." He had been reduced to living on a small savings account he'd managed to put together over the past ten years in addition to VA disability and eventually the Social Security. If he got a job, the Social Security would be cut off. "I'd have to get a job which paid me $500 a month net to make it worthwhile," he pointed out. "And it would have to be a job where I could go on the dialysis machine three times a week. I stay on five or six hours each time. I guess I could do it at night but I do it now during the day."

When I last saw him, he was still waiting for a transplant and trying to manage his life. He said that he really wanted to begin taking some night courses offered at a local community college with the idea of trying to get a teaching job. He had really liked his earlier experience teaching at the fire department.

As our conversation came to an end, he reflected on his condition. "A funny thing about a kidney patient. Everyone of them craves something. I craved gasoline. I would do anything in the world to get gasoline, to sniff it. I finally got off of it, though, thank God, 'cause every time I'd go to get some gas for the car I'd about go outa my head. I talked to several other kidney patients up at the VA, and people craved rocks. They would actually eat pebbles. There was one guy up there who had to have this blanket over his head or he couldn't go, you know, to pee or anything. It was unbelievable. I couldn't figure what was going on."

He continued, comparing himself to others on dialysis he had come to know. "A lot of people, you know, when they find out they've got this disease, I mean, they just give up. That's what the doctors told me, and I guess I've met some. But I want to go back to school and do a lot of things, and I'm going to do them. But there's some people they wheel in up there who can't walk or anything, and they put 'em on the machine and take 'em off and wheel 'em out and they don't do anything. They are just a vegetable. Well, I'm not going to end up like that. I decided, what the devil, if you can't live without it, you gotta live with it. You can't feel sorry for yourself or you're going to kick the bucket."

Mr. Blanton, I've come to realize, is one of the lucky ones. He knew very well, and its been well established generally, that a patient's active participation in dialysis treatment, especially in the rigorous dietary regimen, is critically important for success. Many others, as he came to realize, are unable to achieve that difficult balance between compliance and cooperation, activity and passivity, so needed in dialysis therapy. A common difficulty providers have is finding out how to persuade patients of the need for active participation, how to "reach" and "teach" patients who are severely compromised often in just those abilities needed for persuasion and teaching to work.

For many patients, having end-stage renal disease and being on dialysis are little more than a chronic way of dying. Patients often experience intense despair, depression, even psychosis. Those who, like Mr. Blanton, manage to transcend those psychological difficulties emphasize that they can never forget the physical complications and the omnipresence of death made regularly and starkly clear by what he called "that damned machine." While many patients view the dialysis apparatus as a kind of "miracle" that rescues them from death, they also frequently think of it as a constantly fettering, anthropomorphic presence that takes on a personality of sorts.

Being on dialysis can be volatile. It is a constant reminder of the sheer limits and precariousness of life. Little wonder, then, that patients experience severe mood swings, ups and downs of outlook. Psychiatrist Harry Abrams expressed it lucidly: "In chronic dialysis, the matter is not so much one of eternal life but of living with the rigors of the medical regimen which may bring about what Unamuno termed the 'too long' life."[1] The experience of end-stage renal disease is suffused with complex and paradoxical elements. Without wishing or expecting it, the person's body fails in highly intimate ways: weakness, vertigo, swelling, muscle spasms, nose-bleeding, vomiting, and pain. Quick on the heels of these experiences comes the sudden realization that, as another put it, "even when I am feeling fine, and the machine is running perfectly, and our cat is purring around my feet, and my wife is smiling at me, a thought suddenly runs through my head: 'How did this happen to me?'" Like Mr. Blanton, some patients are able to manage; some learn to cheat cautiously but creatively on the dietary regimen even while they remain haunted by profound body imagery, compelling and inviting reminders of life and loss, with death an always close companion. "I would give a year of my life," one patient once said, "to be able to chug-a-lug a huge schooner of cold, foaming draft beer . . . and another for a whole pitcher of ice water, beaded with little drops of condensation on the outside, cool, crystal clear and a half-gallon deep within . . . but there is no way of forgetting that a kidney machine keeps me alive."

Toward the end of our conversation, Mr. Blanton said that his illness seemed "like a lottery"—one moment you're fine, then suddenly for no reason you start vomiting, all of it "ridiculous bad luck." Yet he was also aware of his "good luck," as are other dialysis patients who manage to stay with the regimen. He remained hopeful and full of plans, for college and teaching. Others are able to continue with their jobs and family lives. These patients are keenly aware of what they often call the "essential factors": the support of my spouse and family; the understanding and cooperation of employers and friends; the nurses, doctors and social workers who not only take care of patients but, as one patient put it, "really care *for* you, so you really feel you can trust them."

The experience of ESRD and of dialysis is critically affected by the presence of caring, supportive people, by the enthusiasm of helpers who are, hopefully, somehow able to understand, listen, and talk about the patient's frightening, debilitating experience. Language, common talk with patients, as I've said several times already, is among the most important therapeutic tools we possess.

But even if the talk is very sensitive to the patient's experience, it can also be devastating. Mr. Blanton, for instance, stressed that he was "shocked, I was really floored, when the doctor told me what I had." No sooner told of his disease and its consequences, Mr. Blanton was also told that the most important thing he must do is to adhere to the dietary restrictions, the dependency imposed by the treatment and the recurrent physical complications associated with dialysis. But, he said, "what gets me more than any of the rest of it is all the things you *can't* do: can't drink this or eat that, and you really wonder sometimes whether it's all worth it."

In the words of another patient, the talk he heard from doctors and nurses about the regimen had another message, one he barely heard at first and came to understand only gradually after much time has passed. Success on dialysis, he said, "requires a strength of character and determination from both the patient and his family." The words doctors and nurses use carry a meaning few patients grasp at first. He came to understand, though, that if he wanted to continue to live, he had to be "strong and determined," he had *to want to live* even while doing so required that punishing set of regimens.

Joe had become keenly aware of this. Toward the end of our conversation, we were interrupted briefly by a nurse who was checking on him. "How're you doing, Mr. Blanton?" she asked straight off.

"Oh, okay, Mary, I guess, and for heaven's sake, please call me 'Joe,'" he responded. "After all, there's little I've got left you haven't seen, you know?" Then he added, "I'd sure like to have a beer right about now. You know, a huge schooner, all frothed up and bubblin', cold as a buck's fanny in mid-winter, and makin' my hand go all numb. Oh, man, would I ever."

"Joe, please," she blurted, "you really just shouldn't keep talking like that. You know you can't do that sort of thing, not any more, not ever. You—"

"Good lord, Mary, *everybody's* been telling me all that sort of thing. That don't keep a man from *thinkin'* about things, you know."

"You'd be so much better off *not* doing even that, Joe. It will only make things more difficult for you when you get home and don't have us to remind you how devastating . . ."

"There's no harm in just thinkin', just kinda, well, you know, dreamin' about such like. Good lord, it's not as if I *want* to—Dr. Zaner, what's the word I'm looking for?"

"You mean you're tempted?"

"Yeh, it's not as if I go around wanting to tempt myself, whatever. The damned thoughts just pop up."

"Well," she replied in her best teacherly manner, "you really should go to a counselor, someone who can help you train yourself to new habits. It's going to be really tough, especially with things like beer and wine and such. That'll keep you off any transplant waiting list, you realize, don't you?"

"The doctor's already gone through all that, so yeh, I guess I understand. Anyway, I wasn't serious just now; just joshing you a bit."

"I understand, Joe, but you've got to realize that things are very serious for you now, that you've got to get used to doing things very differently."

She puttered about some more, straightening the sheets and chiding him, and then left, leaving Joe somewhat depressed in her wake.

"What're you gonna do, doc? I mean, hell, the ideas just keep poppin' up in my head; like, all of a sudden, there it is, that cool, dripping schooner of great beer, just beggin' to be chugged right on down."

"She's right, though, you know?"

"Yeh, I know. Damn! You'd think it was enough just to have your kidneys go out on you; now, a guy's got to change everything, just to stay alive, don't you know? I'm a meat-eater—whoops, I guess I should say I *was* one. But now I can't even sit down to a hamburger, much less a great big, juicy steak all chock full of juice and covered with gravy with a platter full of Vidalia onions. You know what those are, doc?"

"Oh, yes, I've had a few of them."

"No more, I guess, no more."

His voice trailed off, echoes of his plaintive words drifting gently into the now–silent room. His last words as I left still reverberate: "I don't know, doc, that I can do all that, you know? I mean, is it really *worth* it? What've I got ahead? Will I luck out and get a kidney? Will it work? I mean, no more beer, no steak, not even a banana."

Joe's poignant words touched on the other essential thing about the plight of such patients. Even though physicians and nurses are themselves most often focused only on the medical condition and its dietary requirements, what is being said to patients has clear, if also profoundly demanding, moral content. Between the lines, so to speak, his nurse, like his doctor, was telling Joe that he *had* to be strong—morally strong. He had somehow to find in himself that uncommon trait of enduring "grit," of moral courage. And although Joe was feeling much better at the time, he and other patients are given this message very often at a time when they are most deeply affected in their abilities to understand, choose, even to feel and hope beyond the painful immediacy of their present condition and a future that seems more to loom than invite. When patients can understand least well, it seems, the message conveyed is that they must understand most of all. When they are able to think or hope only with great difficulty, they are asked to be at their strongest.

Clearly, to be responsive to the plight of such patients is a venture—not always a happy one—in a kind of moral education. To communicate with them and their families is to embark on a precarious course over terrain that has not been well-explored, that is familiar neither to them nor, oftentimes, to many of the professionals who take care of them. It is a perilous venture that, all things considered, can be well done only if physicians, nurses, families, and others—including ethicists—never forget for a moment just what patients are actually being told.

# If You Don't Ask, You Won't Know

❖

Mrs. French was lying in a bed in the intensive care unit where patients are placed immediately after surgery and recovery from anesthesia. From the nursing station, I could see her—intubated, multiple drips hooked up to her body, writhing in pain. She was awake and alert. Although I couldn't hear what was being said, she was nodding her head, apparently in response to the nurse's questions. It was nothing unusual; in fact, it was all quite common in that unit, so I didn't pay much attention as I was going about one of the rounds my colleagues and I conducted in the unit.

As I was chatting with Susan Ramat, one of the nurses in the unit, she noticed my glance toward Mrs. French's room and asked whether I knew her.

"No, I don't think so; she's new here, isn't she?"

"Oh, yes," Susan replied, "she just came out of surgery earlier this morning."

"Is she alert? She seems to be."

"Well, yes, to an extent anyway. She's still in considerable pain from the surgery, of course."

"I suppose I'd better move on," I said. "Several other units to visit, you know, unless you know of any problems I should know about here."

Susan thought a moment before replying, "No. Everything seems under control today. Oh, did you know about Mr. Mesner over in 34? He's been unconscious for days now, and his family is really having difficulty understanding, coping with it all."

Glancing over to that room, I could see a man lying flat on his back, the usual tubes draping his body and bed. A young woman was standing beside him, looking down. "What's going on?" I asked her.

"That's his niece," Susan said. "She seems to understand. It's his daughter and wife who are having the problems."

"Who's the attending," I wondered out loud. Our protocol requires that we don't get involved with family members without the attending's permission.

"That's one of Dr. Tray's patients, like Mrs. French. He had a bad brain hemorrhage, and it just doesn't seem like he's going to recover."

"I'll call him right away and see if I can be any help. Thanks. But if things get worse, let me know, okay?"

"Sure, Dr. Zaner."

"I'll be back around in an hour or so in any case," I replied.

As I started to walk away, though, Susan mentioned that when I talked with Dr. Tray I might want to ask about Mrs. French, too.

"Oh? Why is that?"

"I'm not altogether sure. I just have a feeling that . . . well, so far as we know, she doesn't have any family, and she's really in a bad way now. Things could get worse, too, in a hurry."

"Really? Why is that?"

"She was brought into a hospital in her hometown with a swollen belly and very high fever, then transferred here for exploratory abdominal surgery. When she was opened up, they found widespread infection. They were able to clean her up a lot, but then discovered an eight-centimeter aneurysm, a triple A, which couldn't be corrected because of all the infection."

An eight-centimeter abdominal aortic aneurysm—good lord, I thought, that's about as big as my fist! "If it breaks or leaks, she's really going to be in bad trouble," I remarked. "And she has no family, at all?"

"Not so far as we know," Susan replied. "The thing is, Dr. Zaner, that she could get into trouble really quickly, and there's just nobody who can speak for her, make decisions, tell us about her wishes, nobody."

"She has no advance directive?"

"Not that we've found," Susan said. "Look in the chart, right there, on the intake form. See? It's left blank where "Living Will" is listed."

"Do you think you or her nurse could ask her about that right now? She seems alert; maybe she could tell us about that. I mean, if she does have a living will, we'd better know about it, right? Even more, if she's signed a Durable Power of Attorney for Health Decisions, we'll have to get ahold of her attorney-in-fact."

Susan walked into Mrs. French's room while I looked over the chart. At one point, I glanced up at the room and could see Mrs. French apparently responding to Susan's questions. The chart wasn't much help. No family members were mentioned. In the place where the form requests the name of the person to be contacted "in the event," a man's name was listed, a William Broadmor. And, as Susan had stated, Mrs. French had experienced high fever and severe pain and tenderness in her stomach. She had gone (or been taken by Mr. Broadmor?) to the local hospital; then, apparently in view of the severity of her condition, she had been transferred to our hospital for surgical evaluation and treatment. Nothing else was in the chart to suggest family members, advance directives, nothing . . . until I got to the surgical permissions form, where it was noted that a "brother" had given permission. *Who is he? Where is he now? Does he know about what's going on now?*

As I was putting the chart down, Susan came back shaking her head: "You never know, do you? She says she *does* have a living will."

"She has one? Where is it?"

"Well, she says that it's at her home."

"Great," I blurted out, "if it's not in a lock-box in a bank, people keep 'em at home, probably hidden away somewhere, too."

"You may be right; all she said was that it's 'at home.'"

"Could you ask her if—let's see, what's his name? Yeh, 'William Broadmor'—if Mr. Broadmor could get it for us?"

"Who's that?" Susan wanted to know.

"He's the one she listed as the person to notify. You're right, no family members are mentioned except a brother, who apparently gave permission for the surgery, apparently by phone?"

"Oh, yes," she replied, "I remember Dr. Tray mentioning that he had called her brother and that he gave permission."

"Didn't he visit?"

"No, so far as we know nobody's visited her, poor lady, and I don't think her brother's been back in touch. I'm not even sure where he lives, but Dr. Tray should know."

Susan went back into Mrs. French's room. As I watched from the nursing station, I could see Mrs. French struggling to reply. Talking while intubated is no easy thing, especially when you're suffering like Mrs. French. Anyway, Susan came back out and told me that Mr. Broadmor was going to find the living will and bring it in.

I was anxious to contact Dr. Tray, too, as he would want to know about the living will. He'd doubtless want to talk with Mr. Broadmor, who, I was thinking, would probably have to be involved in some way if critical decisions had to be faced. Thinking about Mrs. French's "friend," though, I could see some other possible problems on the horizon.

For one thing, many states do not have a "surrogate" statute defining which persons, usually family members, are to be decision-makers in the event an individual loses the ability make his or her own decisions. Although family members are asked to be involved, none of them is the legal surrogate unless one of them is appointed by a court to act as guardian. If there is neither a living will nor a durable power of attorney that names an individual as the legal decision-maker, "attorney-in-fact," and the patient is terminally and irreversibly ill, it is particularly urgent to attend to any conflict or disagreement over what should be done. In fact, if conflicts can't be resolved, the case could easily wind up in court. What concerned me in this instance was the brother: somehow, someone, doubtless Dr. Tray, had found out about him, but there was not a clue I could find that would tell me how he had found out. Dr. Tray had, of course, called for permission, so he would surely know how to get in touch with the brother.

For another thing, when a terminally ill person has no family, or when known family members decline any involvement, and there is no living will or attorney-in-fact, it is important to find out if there is any record at all of the person's wishes. If, as too often happens, there is no such oral or written record, there are real difficulties trying to figure out the best thing to do. Frequently, the medical picture is just not clear enough, which seemed true of Mrs. French, to know for sure that the patient will die even if treatments are continued. But if a person has left some solid indication of what she or he would want done if treatments are futile and doing no more than prolonging death, then it's much easier for physicians and nurses to withdraw supports and focus on comfort and even companionship to terminally ill patients.

One other thing about Mrs. French bothered me: why had she not listed her brother on the form? Were they estranged? How had the surgeon known to call for permission? She was sixty-six years old and had only a brother, who had not visited, so far as was known. On the intake form, only a "friend" was listed. Mr. Broadmor might know Mrs. French very well, but he probably could not help make decisions about her care unless she had actually named him as her attorney-in-fact. Who would know her and her wishes better? On the other hand, suppose his feelings and thoughts about Mrs. French conflicted with her brother's?

As I couldn't resolve any of these questions at the time, when I got back to my office I immediately called Dr. Tray. He was, as it turned out, eager for my involvement and agreed to meet me in about an hour. He also agreed with my suggestion that I put in a long-distance phone call to Mr. Broadmor. When I called, however, Mr. Broadmor told me that he didn't know anything about a living will. "All I know," he said, "is that Dorothy does have a last will and testament, and I am named as the executor. Far as I know, that's all there is. Anyway, when I came in before the surgery . . ."

"You were here?" I asked. "Did you talk to Dr. Tray?"

"Sure, I did, and he wanted to know if there was any next-of-kin, you know, to sign the form for the surgery. Is she alright? Has anything happened? Nobody's called me."

"She's doing okay, Mr. Broadmor, all things considered, but since she's still very sick and Dr. Tray wasn't able to correct everything—that aneurysm especially—"

"Aneurysm?" he blurted out. "She's got an aneurysm, too?"

"You didn't know?"

"No, no, I didn't. I just gave him her brother's phone number up in Ohio, then I had to leave, to get back to work."

"Well, Mr. Broadmor, we really should talk about things. Can you come in for that? And, if you would, Mrs. French indicated that she does have a living will, and this should be put in her chart just in case."

"But if she's doing okay—"

"*Now* she's okay, Mr. Broadmor, but things could change, and it would be very helpful to see what's on the living will. Beyond that, it would be good to know anything else about her and you seem to be very close; after all, she listed your name on the forms here."

"Yeh, well we've been close friends for at least ten years, you know. Far as I know, she's never been in touch with her brother, either. They don't get along. At least, she hardly ever mentions him."

When I asked him whether the people at the first hospital had provided them any information about advance directives, he was a bit vague, though he thought he recalled somebody saying something. Both of them were just so upset, he said, that they weren't paying much attention. We agreed that he would come in the next day and bring in the living will.

I then got back in touch with Dr. Tray. He knew about Mr. Broadmor, of course, and went on to tell me about his call to Mrs. French's brother. "After I got permission on the phone, I asked him if he would be coming down to visit, but he declined. He said that they'd not been close, neither he nor their mother."

"Mother? I hadn't heard about a mother. She must be quite old."

"Oh yes, she's in her late eighties and just suffered a severe stroke, the brother told me. She's unable to talk at all, and from what he said she's pretty much out of it anyway."

"Could we meet this afternoon?" I asked. "I've got a number of questions that need to be cleared up."

We agreed to meet at the nurse's station shortly. When he got there and had gone over my questions, he agreed that in view of Mrs. French's serious condition a call to the brother was appropriate. As we were concluding, Susan Ramat came up with a look at once bemused and concerned.

"Well, wouldn't you know! Mrs. French just indicated that she's got *five children*, three sons and two daughters."

"What?" Dr. Tray's face said it all. "Where in the world are they?"

"Apparently," Susan said, "they all live fairly close to her brother's place in Toledo. But, from what I could gather, they've been at odds for years, don't visit, don't stay in touch . . ."

"*All* of them?" I asked.

"Apparently. But she also mentioned that one of her sons had visited here earlier, several days before the surgery."

"Good heavens," I stammered, "things just keep changing! Do we have any addresses or phone numbers for the children?"

"Not that I can find," Susan stated.

"Well, *I* sure don't have anything in my files," Dr. Tray added. "I had no idea at all, none. Her brother didn't say anything about children, nor did her friend, Mr. Broadmor, say anything either."

We just stood there as the new information sunk in. I mentioned that Mr. Broadmor would be coming in tomorrow and that I'd ask him what he knew. I also pointed out that he had stated, rather matter-of-factly, that Mrs. French and her brother were "not on good terms," that they hadn't seen each other "in years," in fact, not at all during all the time they had known each other.

"Let's just hope," Susan offered, "that nothing goes wrong. She seems to be getting a bit better, anyway."

"Just so long as that aneurysm doesn't act up, she should recover nicely over the next couple of weeks," Dr. Tray pointed out. "There's no reason to expect any problems otherwise."

While we were talking, I took stock of what was known. Mrs. French was doing okay for the present. She had listed her friend as the person to contact "in the event." She stated that she had a living will, but Mr. Broadmor didn't know about that. Her brother had given permission by phone for the surgery and declined to visit, and her friend indicated that the two were estranged. On questioning Mrs. French, Susan had learned of the five children, all adults, and that Mrs. French indicated that she was not close to any of her children. Mr. Broadmor at least knew her brother's phone number, and Dr. Tray was going to call him to find out what he could about the children. Mr. Broadmor was due in tomorrow. For now, then, I thought, all the bases had been covered—except *I* had not yet talked with Mrs. French.

"Do you think it's alright for me to try talking with her now?" I asked.

"It's probably not a good time right now," Susan replied. "She's finally responding to the pain medication and isn't very alert at the moment. Why don't you come by tomorrow morning?" Dr. Tray also thought that would be best. I agreed, and we went our different ways.

Later that day, Dr. Tray called me. He said that her brother confirmed that she had five children, continued to decline to visit, but did give him the phone number of the son who had apparently already visited. "He only came down for an evening, then flew back to Ohio," Dr. Tray said. "Sure wish I had known about that."

"Oh, yeh," I added, "a bunch of questions could have been answered."

"Anyway, I talked with the son. Odd, he didn't seem much

concerned, and said he didn't think another visit could be arranged right away. He did say that I should let him know, though, if things got serious. *'Serious'!* Well . . ."

"Well, you do have his phone number now, at least, and can call him if . . ."

"Yeh, 'if.' Just let me know what Mr. Broadmor has to say, will you? I'll be in surgery most of the morning, but page me anyway. This could be important." Agreeing with him, I hung up.

The next morning, Mrs. French was not doing very well, and was not very responsive when I tried to talk with her. A bit later, Susan paged me to let me know that Mr. Broadmor was in the unit to see me, so I went to meet him. After introductions, we went to the small conference room next to the unit. The living will and her children were foremost on my mind. He immediately pointed out, however, that he couldn't find anything like that. All he knew about, he said, was the last will that she had made several years prior, naming him her executor.

"Any mention in it of her children?"

"Nope, nothing," he replied. "You know, she and her kids haven't seen one another in years. She hardly ever talks about any of 'em, and when she does, it's as if they're strangers. Only thing she's ever said is they don't get along."

"Do they know about you?" I asked.

"Well, I don't know; she's not said anything like that to me, anyway."

"Well, Mr. Broadmor, let me ask: did you take her to the hospital there?"

"Oh, sure; she was really feeling poorly, real bad. She sure couldn't drive herself."

"Did the hospital tell you about advance directives, you know, about living wills and durable powers of attorney for health decisions? You recall I asked you about that when we talked by phone yesterday."

"What? Oh, yeh. Well, I can't rightly say I've ever heard of those things before. Dorothy and me never talked about such like, though, and I just don't think she's signed one of 'em. I think I'd know if she had. Far as I recollect, the folks at the hospital there mentioned something—suppose it could have been what you're talking about, but—and here, too, somebody may have said something, but . . ."

"But she says she has a living will . . ."

"She's probably just confused," he replied, "kinda like me. When you asked on the phone, I thought—and I bet that's what she thought, too—that you meant the last will. I bet that's what she thought."

"Come with me, Mr. Broadmor. Let's go see if she's alert enough to tell us herself, okay?"

We then went back to the unit. He stayed at the nurse's station while Susan and I went in to see her. Still obviously in considerable pain, she was nevertheless sufficiently alert to recognize Susan, who then introduced me. Mrs. French looked at me, questions in her eyes, and I flubbed it, royally.

"Mrs. French, you indicated to Susan yesterday that you have a living will, but your friend, Mr. Broadmor, can't find it at your home, where you said it was . . ." Before I could continue, her eyes recoiled in utter fear. She whipped her head over to Susan on the other side of the bed, pleading, her hands flailing out, tears beginning to brim out.

And Susan, bless her, immediately began soothing, calming, reassuring her that, no, she wasn't dying. Soon, Susan was able to ask her about the living will. Mrs. French again nodded that she did have one. When Susan asked where she kept it, as it wasn't where her friend could find it, Mrs. French managed eventually to indicate that maybe it was with her attorney back in her hometown.

While Susan continued to comfort and reassure her, I slunk out of the room, deeply embarrassed at my blunder. Obviously, I needed to creep up on the question, needed to realize that in her condition *of course* the first thing she'd think about when quizzed about the living will would be *her* death. I just scared her. That it was unintentional was hardly enough. That I had thought that, having already discussed it yesterday, she would of course be able to discuss it today was also a paltry excuse for the blunder, or at least so I saw it.

I managed to relate what had happened to Mr. Broadmor. He knew her attorney and gave me the phone number. I explained and apologized for my blunder. He was kind, then said he'd like to go in to see her. When Susan came out, wondering why I had left the room, I explained to her.

"Nonsense," she said, "she's just having a hard time, and her pain is really awful. I don't think you goofed."

"Well, I do," I replied. "Anyway, I'll get back in to see her later on and apologize for frightening her. Right now, I need to call that attorney and find out about this living will business—finally, I hope!"

I walked out with Mr. Broadmor, continuing to talk about Mrs. French's situation, her children in particular. I pointed out how we had finally found out about them and mentioned that Dr. Tray had learned that her mother was still alive, though not doing well.

"Oh, yes," he replied. "Was he able to talk with her father, too?"

"*Father*? Her father is still alive?"

"Oh, he's real senile, but yes, still alive. Her parents live close to her brother, you know. How about her sister?"

"She has a sister, too? No, none of us here knew anything about that. Do they know that you're the executor of her estate?"

"I suppose so," he said, "but I really don't know, and for that matter don't really care. Dorothy's been by herself for years now, hardly ever in touch with any of that crowd. I'm not sure what's behind it all, but it's clear to me she's not about to have any of them hanging around. When I saw Dorothy today, after you came out, I mentioned that Dr. Tray had talked with her son, Charlie, and she just about went bananas. She just doesn't want him around."

"Well, Mr. Broadmor, you need to know, Mrs. French needs to know, that if she should ever need to have someone else make decisions for her, that will in all likelihood be one of her family, unless she specifically indicates what she herself wants done. That's what advance directives are all about, you know. I'll be in touch with her attorney right away and get a copy of her living will."

"The thing is a lot clearer to me now; as soon as she gets a bit better, maybe you'll help me talk about it with her?"

"Of course."

I said I'd be in touch with him again, and he left the hospital. Okay, stock-taking time again. All that family, all that estrangement. In a way, I thought, it was fortunate that this state doesn't have a surrogate law. If it did, and if Mrs. French didn't have a living will, which would take precedent, she'd be in a real mess, for, as I had said to Mr. Broadmor, one of them would then be responsible for making decisions should she lose that capacity, something that she obviously did not want *at all.*

This situation just kept evolving and changing at every turn. Fortunately, though, she seemed to be recovering. Now, once we had the living will in hand, should things go badly we'd have some guidance. Even so, it seemed to me that at least some of her plentiful family would have to be encouraged to visit; especially now when she was alert and doing fairly well. That way, the potential for disagreements could be probed before any serious issue was present. I made a mental note to discuss the matter with Dr. Tray and went back to my office to call the attorney.

So it goes; you no more get things in hand then they spin out of control again.

"*Who'd* you say? What's the name again?" the attorney asked.

"Mrs. Dorothy French," I repeated. "She indicated that you are her attorney and that you have a copy of her living will in your office."

"I don't think I know the lady," she said.

"But Mr. Broadmor, who's her friend, said you do know her. And Mrs. French said you had a copy of her living will."

"Well, I think I know Bill Broadmor. Just let me look through my files and see what I can find. I'll fax you anything I find, okay?"

"Yes, please fax it to me. Although it's not needed at the present, it's really wise to have it part of her medical chart."

Her attorney did find Mrs. French's file and faxed me a note: "No living will found, only a copy of her last will and testament."

Well, now things could really get difficult, especially if she became worse before we could discuss her wishes with her. The typical procedure, even without a "surrogate" statute, would call for the physician to discuss matters with her family, seek their wishes or, as the case might be, their agreement with the attending's recommendation and go from there. Unless, of course, there were unresolvable disagreements; then, we'd have to advise them that they'd need to have one of them appointed as legal guardian, all of which seemed unfortunate, given what we'd learned about the relationships. Then there was Mr. Broadmor, whom she would doubtless wish to be her decision-maker "in the event." This was all very depressing. In addition to my visit the next morning to apologize to her for what I took to be my blunder, now I'd have to address the whole issue again. *Better take Susan with me,* I thought.

But Susan was not on duty the next day, and this was the first time Mrs. French's current primary nurse had taken care of her. She had in the meantime been extubated, was on "blow-by" (oxygen mask over her nostrils and mouth), and was clearly still experiencing serious pain. But she could talk for herself.

After reintroducing myself—she did not recall meeting me the day before, and didn't know why I apologized—I mentioned that I had talked with Mr. Broadmor.

"What a sweet man, dear Bill," she said.

"He is very concerned about you. Do you recall his visit yesterday?"

"No, my goodness, no; he was here?"

"Yes, Mrs. French, he came in to see you, and he and I were able to have a good talk. He mentioned to me that he would try to get back here within the next couple of days."

"But he has to work, you know, and it's not easy for him to get off. He's got this job; well, it isn't much, but then not many of us old folks, after we retire, can get very much. He can't be taking off just anytime he wants, you know?"

"Are you working, too?"

"Goodness, no, though I really would like to do something useful. Water under the bridge . . ." her voice trailed off, her eyes closing, her face wincing with pain.

"Mrs. French, I called your attorney yesterday. I guess you don't remember now, but you told me that she had a copy of your living will. Do you know what that is?"

"Living will? All I know is that my will is all filled out and Bill's the man. The doctor said I was doing fine, though, so what's all this about my will?"

I went on to describe the directive, why it was important to her, and then mentioned her extensive family. While she remembered that her son had visited her at the hospital, she didn't recall discussing her family with Susan or me yesterday. She made it very clear, though, that she really didn't care one way or the other if any of them visited her, "but I'd as soon they not."

"Did the doctor discuss what he found during the surgery?"

"You mean about the aneurysm?"

"Yes, did he go into that at all with you?"

"Well, yes, he did, just this morning. I know I've got to come back in a while to have more surgery. And he explained why I've got so much medicine to take now—the infection and all—but that it would be some time before I'd be well enough for another operation."

"You realize, then, that you're not yet well, that you've still got a very serious condition?"

"Oh, yes, he made that real clear. Is *that* why you're asking about wills and such?"

"Well, yes, it sure is. I think it's important for you know something, Mrs. French, but you should realize that it's necessary to tread on some sensitive matters, issues you may not feel up to discussing at this point."

"My lord, Dr.—?"

"Zaner, Mrs. French."

"Zaner, then. Okay, I think I know what you're up to: what happens if things don't go well, right?"

"Right, but if you're not up to it now . . ."

"Well, say your piece, and don't beat around the bush."

"Well, Mrs. French, here's the nub of it: if things, as you say, don't go well, now or when you come back for the next surgery, and you're unable to make decisions for yourself, *someone* will have to advise us on your preferences, on what you want the doctors to do."

"You mean, in plain words, if I'm about to die?"

"Mrs. French, in that event—if the aneurysm should burst before you're able to have the surgery done, or if it turns out that it can't be repaired—you really should let your doctors, all of us, know what your wishes are. As it is now, you haven't indicated that. That's what the advance directives are all about: a chance for you to say what you want—that's the living will—or, if you wish, a chance for you to write down *who* you want to make decisions for you—that's the durable power of attorney for health decisions."

"I understand."

"The thing is, Mrs. French, that if you haven't indicated anything, it's normal for your doctors to ask your family, and from what I've heard you say, you'd just as soon they not be involved, is that right?"

"Well, I really don't want that. It's just been so many years, so much has changed."

"I understand. I guess that's why I keep coming here, so that you'll know. And, if I could just mention one other thing."

"Go ahead."

"About your friend, Mr. Broadmor."

"Oh, yes, dear Bill."

"Well, he mentioned that in your last will and testament—that other will—he's named as your executor, is that right?"

"Yes, I wanted him to take care of things."

"Do you also want him to help the doctors make decisions on your behalf, if you're unable to do so yourself?"

"I'm not sure, just not sure. That's such a burden to put on him."

"Well, maybe you need to think about that some. It's probably a good idea, too, to talk with him when he comes back in. If you're feeling up to it, I mean. I'll be happy to discuss all this with him, too, if you want."

"That'd be nice, if it's not too much trouble."

"Mrs. French, that's no trouble; I just want to help out as much as I can. Do you have any questions right now?"

"Fact is, I do, it's just that I'm so beat up."

"Perhaps I should come back later on?"

"It's alright, just give me a moment—well, the thing is, what if something happened before, before—well, if nothing can be done."

"You mean, before you've had a chance to think about the matter?"

"Yes, tonight, or tomorrow morning . . . I really don't want to involve my children or family; we're just too remote, have been for so long."

"You don't need to get into any of those details, Mrs. French, though you certainly may if you wish. I think I understand what you're asking, and I think you really should talk about this with Dr. Tray. He's the one who should know about how you feel, and if you let him know, that's as good as any advance directive. The main thing you need to understand is that he and the rest of us want, and need, to respect your wishes, whatever they may be."

"Well, what I want to say is only that if nothing can be done for me, I don't want any of these tubes and such plugged in, not if there's no point to 'em. And I don't want *anybody* saying otherwise."

"That's what you need to tell Dr. Tray, Mrs. French, even though there's no reason at all right now to think that treatments are pointless. I'll make sure he knows he needs to discuss this with you, and I'll write a note in your medical chart to note the substance of our conversation, so that everyone will know what you've indicated. So will Dr. Tray after you let him know. In the meantime, though, I'll plan on talking with Mr. Broadmor about these matters so that he understands what advance directives are all about, and I'll be visiting with you while you're still here. I want you to know, too, Mrs. French, that everything we've discussed is strictly confidential. Only you, the doctors, the nurses, and me will know anything about this, okay?"

"Oh, I know all that, but I appreciate you telling me."

"One other thing, Mrs. French: I want you know how much I appreciate your willingness to talk with me, and your honesty. I learn a great deal from talking with patients, and feel I should thank you for that. We're all still learning about this kind of thing. Your thoughts and feelings will help me know how to help other people, too."

"Well, that's nice. I appreciate, too, you coming in here and all."

"You're doing fine, and will probably keep on doing fine. I'm sure you'll feel much better by the time I get back in to see you again."

We were able to discuss these matters several times over the course of this hospitalization. Mrs. French did in fact improve considerably and was discharged several weeks later. She's due back for the next surgery, if things continue to go well, in about six months, or sooner if the aneurysm acts up. Before she left the hospital with Bill, we'd been able to discuss the advance directives in some depth. She mentioned that she planned to fill out a living will but needed to think a good deal more about the durable power directive. Bill, it appears, really didn't want to be put in "that position," though he heartily agreed with the idea. He, too, had signed a living will and on my advice had sent copies to his own doctor, the local hospital, and even our hospital, following Mrs. French's example.

The way this situation evolved was a bit unusual, for in very few does vital information become known like this one. Since it happened rather recently, I was able to recall its ins and outs in more detail than others. However unusual, the way things developed harbors some important clues about the way ethical issues emerge. From thinking that she had "no family" but that she did have a "living will," we learned over the span of a mere three days that she *did* indeed have a family and *no* living will. None of this would have been known if she hadn't been asked. If you don't ask, you'll never know. In some cases, you won't know about matters that may turn out to be terribly vital to the patient and others who are immediately involved in caring for her. Not that asking is easy; far from it. I learned that well during my first two visits with Mrs. French.

More than that, though, was significant to this case. When patients are not capable of making their own decisions, providers invariably turn to families, even when this is not legally required. That is both natural and understandable. With some, however, that could be precisely the wrong thing to do, and for many different reasons. Some people point out that their families just don't know them any longer; others that family members would be too deeply affected by having to make, or even help to make, key medical decisions. Still others say that they have become so deeply estranged from their families that they are adamantly opposed to any of them having anything whatever to do with them, especially important medical decisions. In any case, of course, the same rule applies: if you don't ask and probe, even when it becomes decidedly uncomfortable, you won't know.

# Afterword

Albert Schweitzer once emphasized that in each of us is a moral sense that, though usually dormant, can be brought to the surface on special occasions. Each of the situations portrayed in these narratives is precisely that kind of special occasion. Each of them confronts the people involved—and ourselves, to the extent that we can feel the difficult issues these people faced—with a basic challenge to their sense of self. What and who we are, what we hope to be and become, even whether we will continue to be at all, is in one way or another at stake in these circumstances. This poses basic moral questions.

I think especially about recent developments in genetics—what it harbors for us, for what we must come to understand by moral life—and I keep returning to Mrs. Blackman's situation. What we need is a different way of thinking about what is good, right, and fair, as we need to appreciate how our promising discoveries place us willy-nilly in the embrace of wholly new choices and new forms of responsibility. What might these be? What resources do we have to grapple with those terribly complex issues? But those aren't, by any stretch, the only issues we face; we need only think about those other situations, each of which presents its own sort of puzzles and problems. What resources do we have to help us deal with them?

All of the people in these narratives, however, are involved in critical situations that appeal for—even demand—resolution, and there is no way for us to get on about our lives without somehow responding. Whether we or someone we care for is gravely ill, we undergo that difficult but unavoidable experience of finding ourselves challenged, of having to face basic moral questions. We experience the unavoidable need to respond. We must reach decisions for which we are responsible, decisions that involve consequences with which we then have to live.

One way to think about this is to consider what happens when we face a *problem*. Problem has a Greek etiology, *problēma*, which has two usages: it can denote either a shelter or an obstacle, suggesting a common root—something that juts out. A large boulder juts out on a mountain path, for instance, and can serve either as protection or hindrance, sanctuary or obstruction. Whether it is one or the other, of course, is directly connected to what we are doing at the time we encounter it.

Clearly, it is the sense of obstacle that has been handed down as the primary meaning of our word, "problem." It is something that needs to be resolved, a disturbance that needs to be settled. Whatever it may be that we confront as a problem, we need to get around it, go over it, or smash through it somehow—only so long as we want or need to continue going on that blocked path. Of course, if we decide that continuing is not worth the effort needed to settle things, everything can be solved rather simply: change our course, go in a different direction. Although the thing is still there, it is then no longer *in our way*. Having decided to go elsewhere, we no longer find the obstacle to be a problem.

But if it is important to keep going that way, we've got the problem. We cannot continue without doing something about what has blocked our way (whether illness, marital difficulties, a recalcitrant child). A "boulder" of some sort stands there blocking the way and demands attention and some kind of resolution. Note that some things won't work. We can't keep doing what we were doing, like pretending we're still healthy and denying there are any problems with our marriage or that our child is really doing fine; for that is just what got us to the obstacle in the first place, and we'd merely keep bumping up against it again. Coming across the obstacle, we must to do something *different* to find a solution. We have reached what was described by Plato as an *a-poría,* an acute impasse. What must we do to resolve the dilemma?

The couple whose fetus was found to have congenital anomalies, the parents whose baby was inevitably going to die, the young man who refused dialysis, the wife whose husband wouldn't take the genetic test—all of them, and the others in these stories, faced an *a-poría*, a pressing impasse that, at the same time, raised distressing moral problems and called on their moral resources in order to resolve them. None of these people had an easy time. Far from it. Each had to decide (literally, "to cut off from," *de-caedere*) the temporal course of events by choosing one alternative and thus cutting off the others. (Even if the decision were not to decide, that's still a decision.) How did these people make these decisions? How did they then live with the aftermaths?

In a sense, it's clear that some of them simply had no choice, at least no easy one. The circumstances they faced when I became involved reflected early decisions in which some options had already been closed off by the course of events. Johnny, for instance, was going to die no matter what. The only decision left, it seemed, was where and with whom, in the hospital with the nurses and doctors or at home with parents? Like Johnny's parents and providers, all of the people in these cases were confronted with circumstances that were irreversible, and the press of time and medical condition had closed off many options. Joe Blanton, too, had to face a stark fact about himself: he could no longer do or be what he wanted, not even regarding his daily meals; he had to change, unavoidably and basically, who and what he was. So, too, did Mrs. French have to face the reality of her own bodily limitations, not only the peritonitis, but, not too far off, the prospect of having additional surgery to correct the abdominal aneurysm. And, in the meantime, she had to make some troubling decisions about her estranged family and her close friend, Bill.

If only by hindsight, all these people faced situations with few, if any, choices—or at least the alternatives available to them were very limited. It is just this makes their situations so compelling. For the couple with the compromised fetus, for instance, as time went on, options faded, and everyone involved seemed all the more drawn to them. Even at the beginning of his life, Johnny's remaining gut was so tiny and fragile that surgery offered only a small chance of help, but enough to prompt everyone to go with it, to have the surgery even while they knew, or suspected, all along that the odds were very much against them and would in any case leave few choices along the way. Much hope, but few decisions—this describes each person's own history, experiences, beliefs, values, and medical condition.

Yet at some point, as each case unfolded, each of them did face a decision, even if it meant only deciding to recognize and accept the inevitable and somehow martial their inner resources as they faced having to live with the aftermaths. Joe Blanton, for instance, faced not only his devastating disease but the painful reality of costs, insurance, and planning some kind of future for himself. Or, think about that man whose developing fetus tested positive for the genetic disease. What should he now do? And about his wife, how can she now manage? How do they make decisions? How do people manage to live with crises like these? What resources do they call on? Could Mrs. French really ask her close friend, and not her family, to be her decision-maker should she require someone to make decisions for her?

Understanding these issues requires recognizing that the problems and impasses were posed by the circumstances these people faced. The impasses themselves called for choices, decisions. As an *appeal* for a *response*, each situation is tied to specific circumstances, even though these and the problems they posed may not have been clearly understood, or even recognized as such. But the problems are present and pressing even if a person fails or refuses to acknowledge them or denies what's going on.

While Mrs. Blackman seemed to understand very well what she and her husband had to confront now and in the future, he remained adamant in refusing to acknowledge that there was a problem. He was, perhaps, in a kind of denial—perfectly understandable, since the results of the genetic test harbored serious implications for him, his wife, his offspring, and others in his family and kindred. Everything in their situation was oriented by certain facts, actual and suspected. There was the prospect of his having the flawed gene and passing it on to his child; her acute sense of the unfairness of it all; her having to face whether to tell him and whether to abort, and then his finding out anyway. While his wife's appeal to him to have the test went unheeded, it was surely not unheard. The appeal—more accurately, perhaps, the *demand*—implicit to these facts, especially the eventual abortion and divorce, did elicit a response, albeit not the one either of them in any way wanted. Think only about what she faced after the results came back positive: her developing fetus did indeed have the faulty gene, which meant that her husband also had it and at some future point he would begin showing symptoms and soon after would become increasingly demented and debilitated until death within a few years. Her dilemma is *compelling*. Realizing the circumstances she faced, we feel *drawn* to her, to her developing baby, and to her husband.

And don't we feel much the same sort of feeling of *being drawn to the others*? Surely Mrs. Albert felt herself drawn to the budding life still in her womb and facing disaster, or else she could not have so vividly imagined its doomed future, seeing it as "wrong" to force her baby to live like that. Or consider how compelling Johnny's story is, or that of his parents. Despite early appearances, they were drawn to him during his remaining days. The same was true for his nurses, who were so deeply bonded to him that their difficulty in letting go was almost palpable.

Recall Mr. Redstone's ex-wife, Sally. Despite being divorced, she was willing, even eager, to be with him during the exceedingly hard days of waiting for a transplant. Then, should a lung be found for him, she agreed to be with him through the surgery and afterward for who knows how long? We are forcefully drawn to them in their circumstances. Then there is that elderly woman who held off dying so that she could be with her children and her old friend one last time, and the dialysis patient's mother who wanted desperately for his refusal of dialysis to be respected yet did not want him to die as a result. Although Tom muted his feelings during our early conversations, it became perfectly obvious that he did not want to hurt his mother by his adamant refusal to have dialysis. We sense how deeply Tom felt torn away from what he had most wanted to be, compellingly pulled to keep alive his hope for independence even while he thought it was lost, as dead as he thought he now wanted to be. But it was not death, but a particular way of being alive that he most wanted. If we contrast this case with Joe Blanton's, moreover, it's clear how much we have to recognize and appreciate the specific circumstances of each individual. Joe all along wanted so much not only to live but to live in quality ways—to go back to school, to become a teacher—while Tom's vision was at first so clouded.

Listening to Mrs. French, realizing just what she not only had just gone through but what she still had to face, you can't help but be drawn to her, wanting somehow to help. Could, or should, anything be done about her family? Why were they so estranged from each other? And her friend, Bill, a gentle, caring man who had become so close to her, knew her and what she would want better than anybody else yet seemed unable to handle the onerous task of being her decision-maker should she lose that capacity.

Being with these people, it's impossible to remain at a distance. Even meeting them through their stories, our tendency to be disinterested, to take their stories as just stories, is canceled. Instead, we feel compelled to *notice* the moral issues being faced by severely ill, threatened, or dying patients. It's as if we *cannot* pass them by; we are drawn to them at the deepest level of our own moral being, as if, in Schweitzer's lucid words, a moral sense were awakened despite ourselves.

Turning to another person, adverting to or noticing the other, was termed *Du-Einstellung* by Alfred Schutz. What he meant can be

seen if we consider William Golding's novel *Lord of the Flies.* A group
of children are marooned on an island during wartime and are formed
into a little society (a veritable Leviathan) by the clever, devious Jack.
Kept in check by his rigid rules, the children perform rituals to
placate what Jack wants them to believe is a "beast," the "lord of the
flies," or Beelzebub, which they pacify with the gift of a pig's head
on a stake. After an almost mystical encounter with this "lord," one
of the boys, Simon, makes his way slowly and painfully through
creepers and thickets, over sharp rocks, up the cliff to the top of the
hill where the beast was seen. He reaches the top and, buffeted by the
wind, sees "a humped thing suddenly sit up on the top and look down
at him"—*the beast.* Hiding his face, he moves closer and sees a
corpulent figure bow forward; then he understands. It is a man whose
parachute has been hung in the high rocks, and as the wind catches
the chute it flails out the man's limbs, the beast is nothing but that.
His first reaction is to examine these "colours of corruption" held
together by the layers of rubber and canvas. The putrid odor is too
much, and he vomits. Then, feeling pity for the "poor body that
should be rotting away," he frees the parachute lines "and the figure
from the wind's indignity." Why pity? Why does he feel drawn to
restore dignity to a putrid corpse?

Surveying the scene on the beach below, he sees that the boys
have moved their camp away from the hill's base. Then, drawn "to the
poor broken thing that sat stinking by his side," he realizes that "the
beast was harmless and horrible; and the news must reach the others
as soon as possible." He is drawn to the others. He knows that things
have become terribly wrong with the other children, that the "beast"
had been used by Jack to form them into a menacing gang. He wants
to set things right, to tell the truth about the beast. He also knows
full well what is bound to happen to him when he goes back among
them, for he has already clashed with Jack and seen what he did to
other children when they confronted him. Yet down he goes. It is
already night. The boys have been whipped into a frenzy by Jack.
"Kill the beast! Cut his throat! Spill his blood!" A storm on the
horizon shatters the sky. A "throb and stamp of a single organism,"

the boys suddenly see a thing crawling out of the forest. "Him! Him!" they shout and set upon it with sticks, beating and crunching its bones, biting and tearing its flesh. At the last moment, they hear it cry out "against the abominable noise something about a body on the hill."

Ultimately, Simon's compulsion to tell the truth to the other children results in his death; he is mistaken for the monster. That powerful and devastating outcome is integral to Golding's tale. But what fascinates me even more is when Simon is still up on the hill and learns the truth about the monster, his experience of feeling drawn to others, his deep sense of compassion for the other children. Indeed, he even understands that the pilot's corpse is not simply something dead and gone, but is a haunting reminder of that person, a person who still deserves respect and should be treated with dignity.

The people in these narratives speak of the same thing— something, I think, about moral life. Listening to these people, I hear a compelling theme centering around the feeling of compassion for those people with whom we are always in some type of significant relationship. At times, being with others is profoundly simple. The simple act of *being* at the bedside of a dying person may be all that one can do, and that is precisely what is needed to affirm our common humanity. To witness the sick or maimed is, as Schweitzer noted, to experience an appeal, to have an otherwise dormant moral awareness awakened, most immediately felt as the need to respond, to let them know they matter to us and, in that sense, that they are cared for.

We can see this more when we look at things from the sick person's point of view. People who are sick or injured not only want to know what's wrong, why they're hurting, what can be expected, what can and should be done about it, but they also want to know whether anybody *cares*, whether the people who *take* care *of* them also care *for* them. With the dying person, these complex feelings are even more revealing. Some people are haunted by whether or not their lives made any difference, whether they mattered. Others want especially to let us know they care for us, that we who remain alive matter to them, that our lives have been worthy.

To come across this phenomenon of *worth* is to learn something very significant about ourselves. We *are enabled to be* what we are only within these complex and mutual relationships with others, relationships which voice that complex and often troubled imperative. We need and want other people to know that each of us is important, and we need and want to know that we matter to them. It has been noted often enough that when we are born, we are old enough to die. But when we are born, we surely *will* die unless we are nurtured and tended by others, most obviously by our parents. We owe our very lives to other people, and from birth on we exist within multiple and complex relationships, bonds, and ties.

It is true enough that we are not connected with everyone in the same way or to the same intensity. Not everyone's view of us matters to the same degree, although it should also be pointed out that there are times—especially for people in hospitals who are seriously sick or dying—when it can be terribly important for simply *anyone* to take notice, pay attention, listen. As our relationships with other people vary, so do our individual experiences of illness. What is serious for one may not be for another; one person's acute pain may be merely discomfort for another. Still, the experiences of illness in these stories include a dimension of foreboding, a sense of actual or impending loss with grief and mourning coloring every moment. In this, Alfred Schutz was on target in observing that every moment of our waking lives is haunted by a "fundamental anxiety" that ultimately each of us will die.

To experience illness is to experience that underlying sense of limit, of uncertainty and finitude. This "fear of death," as it is sometimes called, is more complex than usually thought, for it is textured by that deeply personal need for being noticed and heeded, for *mattering* to other people—at times those who are intimately known by the person, at other times simply anybody who happens to be there. And to be present with the sick or maimed is to find and feel oneself *called on.* Just here, one sees the real significance of plain talk, a simple touch, the direct look and the sick person's need to hear that word, feel that touch, note that look. That simple human touch, the sound of the human voice, the notice in the human look appear as touchstones of the moral order and enable the person to know in the most immediate way that he or she is recognized and affirmed. This act of affirming of one another, of being with one another in our mutual relatedness, is the hearthstone of our common humanity.

We know this best and most pervasively in our daily lives. We want a friend to appreciate why we plan on doing something that may seem out of character, and we blurt out "but put yourself in my shoes!" Or someone appeals to us to put ourselves in her shoes, to look at things from within her life and concerns. If we do, if we for the moment cease viewing things from our own set of concerns and look at things from her point of view, maybe then we'll understand why doing what she plans makes sense *to her*. Even if we wouldn't ever do what she's planning to do, maybe we'll appreciate why she wants to do it.

I have called this act of appreciating one another, of being drawn to others who ask us to see things from their points of view, "affiliation." When we do this, we sense the need to feel things as they feel them. Just that, I believe, is what happened to me while being with the people in these stories. Just that is what they urgently wanted us to feel. Just that is what it means *to care for* sick people while trying to take care of them. To respect sick people is to affiliate with them. To affiliate is to undergo this feeling with other people, to have *compassion*—an experience that has a number of different forms. Listening to a critically ill patient and talking with patients, indeed, even the simple act of touching, can embody this "feeling-with-others." Feeling compassion is a key part of learning to think and deliberate ethically. One physician states this lucidly: "the entree into the world of the sick person," Arthur Kleinman says, is to put ourselves "in the lived experience of the patient's illness . . . family members and important people in the wider social circle."[1]

Being in these situations, I often felt as if I were a sort of reminder of things that might otherwise be forgotten in the press of events. Introducing myself as "an ethicist" seemed to prompt many of these people to think about things that were otherwise likely to be left unsaid, often even to one another. In a sense, to be seen as someone concerned with ethics is to be the person who affirms that talking about these issues, however they may be individually defined or understood, is important. Perhaps the reason for this is that most of us usually don't have to think about our own most basic beliefs. We are rarely inclined to do so, and events in our daily lives don't usually oblige us to serious reflection. Indeed, few of us are used to the self-reflection that serious moral challenges force us to undergo. Being inexperienced, we find these situations chilling and frightening. Many people are shattered by the personal crises brought on by serious affliction to ourselves or to those we love. To come on the scene as an ethicist is not only to be a reminder of that need for deliberation about deeply serious issues, but is also to serve as an affirmation of that need and the significance of those issues and the profound feelings they evoke. It is not merely "okay" to consider how we feel about terminating life supports, about abortion, or about people who won't cooperate; those issues are precisely what *must* be thought about. To serve as an ethicist is to be the occasion for these people—patients, families, friends, doctors, nurses, and other providers—to undergo the disquiet and hardship of reflection and deliberation. Situations involving illness or injury are compelling. Everyone involved in clinical encounters sooner or later realizes that they must think about what one feels is most precious, most hoped for, and most worthwhile in life.

Becoming involved in ethics under these circumstances, we are quickly drawn into these very issues, having to focus on those multiple, complex relationships—most immediately, that dyadic relationship between the primary providers and the patient/family. More concretely, the ethicist's involvement is the occasion for highly specific talk among just *these* individuals with just *their* lives, circumstances, concerns, feelings, aims, and proposals for acting. The circumstances are *theirs*, not mine, as are the issues, options, decisions, and the outcomes. My role is *not* to try and figure out what was right or what these people should do, nor is it to make a guess about what I would do as if I was the one on the spot, for few if any of us really knows what we might do were we so involved.

It seemed to me that what I could do was help them think about what was at stake for each of them as carefully and fully as time and circumstances allowed and as much as possible within the frameworks of their respective beliefs. This involved exploring matters that were invariably very difficult to get to and discuss, much less to figure out what course of action seemed most congruent with their respective beliefs. Few of these people had ever been called on to do this kind of probing. They were neither by habit inclined to do this, nor had issues arisen in their lives that forced them to deliberate about what was most basic, most worthwhile of all things. The problems they faced, of course, did exactly that. With the stakes so high—in many instances, life itself—it was imperative for them to consider those issues. Not having done it before, or at least not having done it to any great extent before, made it not only difficult but disturbing.

It was a remarkable experience to be with each of these people during these times. Each of them wanted desperately to do the "right" thing, to be "good" and "just" in facing really awesome problems. And most of them did so with impressive courage. But, as we all know, *wanting* to do the "right," the "good," and the "just" and *knowing* what these mean are two very different things. Wanting is simply not enough, not in the face of the sort of problems they each faced. Each person wanted to know just what the right, the good, and the just were.

What was remarkable to me—beyond each person's earnest desire to know and to act in the best way and the courage it took to tackle that—was that as each case evolved, as talking and listening went on, decisions often as not seemed somehow just to emerge. I almost want say that they came about naturally, yet that's not quite on target, since it doesn't capture the real struggle each of them went through nor the passion with which they went at it. Yet, through those conversations, those dialogs, people seem somehow to come across ways of resolving their problems, dilemmas, and enigmas.

This process of arriving at or discovering decisions was lucidly suggested by sociologist Kurt Wolff when he was trying to describe what I take to be very much the same thing, but in a rather different connection. At crucial times in our lives, during crises when we are seemingly at a loss to know what to do, we are often as not grabbed by an idea. "What has to be done" seems somehow to catch us. It's almost as if we are caught by it than that we have discovered it ourselves. Just this occurs to Simon in Golding's novel: having come upon the truth of the "beast," not only must dignity be restored to the dead parachutist but "the others must be told!" What must be done seems somehow to pop up, though where it comes from we are at a loss to say.

Wherever it comes from, the decision often seems to dawn on us, to catch us. If we can just get ourselves in the right frame of mind to give into it, why, then there it is. This notion of "catch," of "being caught" by a notion, comes from the Latin word *invenire,* which literally means "to come upon." When something occurs to me, it "comes over me"; I am beset by it. What "comes out" of what occurs to us may be a decision, a poem, a painting, or even clarity in an urgent question. As Wolff points out, when something like this happens, when a decision or clarity bubbles up and is suddenly there for us, not only has something "come out," been "invented," but we ourselves have also "come upon," been "invented."[2] As when we make something: creating it, we find that we've also been creating ourselves and are thereby changed by the experience.

Just this is what struck me time and again while being with each of these people. When the dialysis patient, Tom, for instance, began talking about his job and his hopes of getting an apartment, a veritable transformation took place in his gestures and words. I could almost see a light bulb go on. He was suddenly enlivened, talking about how he would get back to work, get an apartment. Yet only a moment before, he had been muted, his gestures slow and heavy, his voice and words softened by sadness, grief, loss.

I'm not quite sure just what to make of this process. Several things seem involved. On the one hand, the process seems closely tied in with an internal spiritual struggle. On the other, other people often play a key role in that struggle. Talking with Tom afterward, I think I got a glimpse of it. If I said something directly about what he had been through, he seemed puzzled, as if he didn't quite understand what I was driving at. But when we talked of other things, walked around the topic indirectly, the real issues he faced seemed to bubble up of their own accord. For instance, when I mentioned that one of the things I do in my job is to teach medical students and suggested he might be helpful in the effort to sensitize them to patients like himself, he was at first surprised. As we talked about it, he suddenly noted, almost as if to himself, how important it was for him to have the chance simply to "talk about things," to have someone willing just to listen.

As I think about this now, having that chance to take the lead in our discussion, and to listen to Tom seems very important. At first I had tried very directly to get to what I thought were important issues: death, his mother, etc. What I hadn't realized is that, while it's doubtless true that he had not really thought about the implications of what his refusal *meant*, he had been *living with* the refusal and its implications. In a sense, he knew full well what was going on and what he was doing. But it was only when, a bit frustrated that I couldn't get him very worked up about discussing his situation, we began talking about him—his life, his hopes, his frustrations, his plans—that everything came pouring out. It was as if the talk about other things was a way of talking about what he needed, and really wanted, to talk about.

The *indirection* here strikes me as significant. Living with serious issues, suffering from all they imply, can get to be just too much. We get a belly full of dwelling on that and just can't find a way out. It's as if we are just too wrapped up in things and need help somehow to get out in order to get another perspective. But that can't be done, for what we face is just so awful, so critical, that thinking about other things seems quite impossible. Now bring in another person willing and able to just be there, to listen, and to talk about little things.

Sometimes we have a kind of "Ah-ha!" experience and sudden insight happens to us, at which point direct talk finally becomes possible.

Working in clinical ethics seems to serve pretty much that role: helping people who must make decisions to think deeply about their own beliefs and values and to understand what issues their circumstances pose for them and how they might best face them. At the same time, people in clinical ethics have to promote not only these conversations, but must keep them *focused* on the moral facets of their lives from within the circumstances and problems posed to these people. Ethicists are rather like readers and interpreters of obscure texts. They help to identify, in the midst of complex relationships and clinical problems, just what needs specific notice and attention. Within the gradually unfolding moral perspectives of the primary decision-makers, ethicists help pick out key decision points and options. They help people go through their options and possible outcomes in the light of their own concerns and values, finding what seems most reasonable for them. As the meaning of obscure texts rarely jumps out and announces itself to the reader, the ethicist has to become a sort of detective, collecting and probing clues and hints, most often nestled within an inevitable bristle of emotions. They then hold them up for inspection and help these people test them to see if they make sense, are viable, and stand up to the test. For this, especially because of the emotions that so texture such clinical situations when the stakes are high and people are desperate, ethicists have to learn never to take anything for granted. At every point they must put themselves in the shoes of those who face the grievous problems. If, as a physician friend of mine likes to insist, language is *one* of the most important tools of medicine, language is the *only tool* for the ethicist, the only tool for helping people reflect on every facet of their situation.

Being with people facing personal crises has had a real impact on how I understand myself and, of equal importance, how I understand my profession as a philosopher. It has made the ancient Socratic practice of engaging people where they actually live—in the "marketplaces" of civic and personal life—ring with clarion tones. Philosophy was never a merely academic exercise for me, but working in hospitals and clinics has made *practicing* philosophy a vivid reality. Perhaps this book will also help others in my profession appreciate the pressing need to be involved with people and to help them with their problems in the contexts where they actually occur.

Listening to people tell their stories, their triumphs and tragedies, seems to me to be the best way to understand the human dimensions of the problems we increasingly face during times of illness and injury. Maybe these stories will help other people come to a richer understanding of the problems and difficulties faced by the people in these narratives. I also hope that in reading and thinking about these people, you, the readers, will be helped in grappling with times when, as is inevitable, you find yourselves in difficult straits facing awesome decisions that try all our souls and challenge us to courage and honesty with ourselves.

# Notes

## FOREWORD

1. Richard M. Zaner, *The Way of Phenomenology* (New York: Western Publishing Company, 1970).

2. Ibid., 25.

3. Ibid.

## CHAPTER 1

1. Eric J. Cassell, *Talking With Patients,* vol. 1 (Cambridge: MIT Press, 1985), 119.

## CHAPTER 3

1. About a year prior, one had been established at a local private hospital through the Center for Clinical-Medical Ethics at the University of Chicago, headed by Dr. Mark Siegler.

2. As we all realize, conversations like this occur all the time, especially in contexts where people are confronted with critical and deeply difficult decisions. A most perceptive psychiatrist, R. D. Laing, has drawn wonderfully apt attention to this sort of "knot" or "whirligog" in his fascinating study *Knots* ([New York: Pantheon Books, 1970], 5, 75).

3. I use these and several others from Laing's study *Knots* to help me think about just these sorts of complexities of interpersonal relationships in my *The Context of Self* (Athens: Ohio University Press, 1981), 238-41.

## CHAPTER 6

1. Prenatal diagnostic procedures are truly a "growth industry," especially over the past decade, and new procedures are continually being added to the list. *Chorionic villus sampling,* which can be performed as early as eight-weeks gestational age, involves studying cells taken from the villi on the outermost extraembryonic membrane; *amniocentesis* is the surgical transabdominal perforation of the uterus to obtain amniotic fluid; *fetoscopy* is used to view the fetus *in utero* by means of a fetoscope; *ultrasonography* is the visualization of the fetus *in utero* by recording the reflections of echoes of pulses of ultrasonic waves. Each of these procedures enables the detection of a variety of problems.

## CHAPTER 9

1. Harry S. Abrams, "Psychological Dilemmas of Medical Progress," *Psychiatry in Medicine* 3 (1972): 56.

## AFTERWORD

1. Arthur Kleinman, *The Illness Narratives* (New York: Basic Books, 1988), 232-33.

2. Kurt Wolff, *Surrender and Catch* (Boston: D. Reidel, 1976), 21-22, 33, 195.

# Suggested Reading

Baird, Joseph L., and Deborah S. Workman. *Toward Solomon's Mountain: The Experience of Disability in Poetry.* Philadelphia: Temple University Press, 1986.

Becker, Ernest. *The Denial of Death.* New York: The Free Press, 1973.

Bishop, Anne H., and John R. Scudder, Jr. *Nursing: The Practice of Caring.* New York: National League for Nursing Press, 1991.

Bishop, Jerry E., and Michael Waldholz. *Genome.* New York: Simon and Schuster, 1990.

Bosk, Charles L. *Forgive and Remember: Managing Medical Failure.* Chicago and London: University of Chicago Press, 1979.

Cassell, Eric J. *The Nature of Suffering and the Aims of Medicine.* New York and London: Oxford University Press, 1991.

Hardy, Robert C. *Sick: How People Feel About Being Sick and What They think of Those Who Care for Them.* Chicago: Teach'em, Inc., 1978.

Hunter, Kathryn Montgomery. *Doctors' Stories: The Narrative Structure of Medical Knowledge.* Princeton: Princeton University Press, 1991.

Katz, Jay. *The Silent World of Doctor and Patient.* New York: The Free Press, 1984.

Kleinman, Arthur. *The Illness Narratives: Suffering, Healing and the Human Condition.* New York: Basic Books, 1988.

Laing, R. D. *Knots.* New York: Pantheon Books, 1970.

Pellegrino, Edmund D. *Humanism and the Physician.* Knoxville: The University of Tennessee Press, 1979.

Sacks, Oliver. *The Man Who Mistook His Wife for Hat, and Other Clinical Tales.* New York: Harper and Row, 1987.

Van den Berg, Jan Hendrick. *Medical Power and Medical Ethics.* New York: W. W. Norton, 1978.

Zaner, Richard M. *Ethics and the Clinical Encounter.* New York: Prentice-Hall, 1988.

# Index